Natural Alternatives

to Prozac

Also by Michael Murray

Encyclopedia of Natural Medicine
Natural Alternatives to Over-the-Counter and Prescription Drugs
The Healing Power of Herbs
Natural Alternatives for Weight Loss

THE GETTING WELL NATURALLY SERIES
Arthritis
Chronic Fatigue Syndrome
Diabetes and Hypoglycemia
Male Sexual Vitality
Menopause
Stress, Anxiety, and Insomnia

Natural Alternatives to Prozac

Michael T. Murray, N.D.

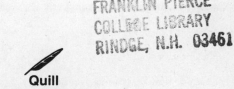

Quill
William Morrow
New York

IMPORTANT: PLEASE READ

The information in this book is intended to increase your knowledge about natural remedies and by no means is intended to diagnose or treat an individual's health problems or ailments. The information given is not medical advice nor is it presented as a course of personalized treatment. There may be risks involved in connection with some of the natural remedies suggested in this book, just as there may be risks involved in connection with prescription drugs. Therefore, before starting any type of natural remedy or medical treatment, or before discontinuing any course of medical treatment you may now be undergoing, you should consult your own health-care practitioner.

The Library of Congress has cataloged a previous edition of this title.

Library of Congress Cataloging-in-Publication Data

Murray, Michael T.
 Natural alternatives to prozac / Michael T. Murray.
  p. cm.
 Includes bibliographical references and index.
 ISBN 0-688-14684-8
  1. Depression, Mental—Alternative treatment. 2. Depression,
 Mental—Nutritional aspects. I. Title.
 RC537.M867 1996
 616.85'27—dc20   95-47489
                CIP

Paperback ISBN 0-688-16628-8

Printed in the United States of America

First Quill Edition 1999

1 2 3 4 5 6 7 8 9 10

BOOK DESIGN BY LAURA HAMMOND HOUGH

www.williammorrow.com

Preface

Depression is a major problem in the United States. Nearly fifteen million Americans will suffer true clinical depression each year. Depression is also a big business for drug companies, especially for the maker of Prozac—Eli Lilly and Company. It is now estimated that more than twelve million people around the globe (including more than six million Americans) take Prozac, resulting in yearly sales of over $2 billion for Eli Lilly and Company. Is Prozac the answer to the growing epidemic of depression? No. There are natural alternatives to Prozac that are safer and more effective.

Why aren't these natural measures as popular as Prozac? Our current medical system is largely controlled by the pharmaceutical industry. The drug companies have the money and the power to mold medical thought. The popular treatment of psychological disorders with drugs is a prime example of the influence that the pharmaceutical industry has on medical practice. An editorial that appeared in the medical journal *Biological Psychiatry* summarized this influence and what comes with it:

"The overall influence of the industry is to emphasize drug treatment at the expense of other modalities: psychotherapy, social approaches, nutritional, herbal, and natural remedies, rehabilitation, general hygienic measures, nonpatentable drugs, or other alternative approaches. It focuses attention on disorders that are treatable by drugs, and may promote over diagnosis. It reinforces the practice of dealing with disease by treatment of symptoms, and diverts interest from prevention."

The whole blame for the popularity of antidepressant drugs cannot be cast on the pharmaceutical industry. It is much easier for doctors to write out a prescription than to try to seek out underlying psychological or physiological factors. Our society as a whole has become composed of individuals who have become dependent upon the quick fix of modern pharmacy. Too often the cost of this instant gratification is side effects. With Prozac the side effects can be dangerous.

Depression is not caused by a physiological deficiency of Prozac. Although it is in vogue to refer to people as "Prozac deprived," the human brain does not require Prozac to function properly. While Prozac and other antidepressants are often effective in elevating mood and reducing depression and anxiety, the downside is that they tend simply to mask symptoms and do not address the underlying cause. This effect is common with many common drugs.

An effective treatment of any psychological or physical condition should be focused on addressing the cause rather than the symptom. In this book I have detailed measures that can eliminate depression and raise moods safely and effectively without taking antidepressant drugs such as Prozac.

I believe that in the future, drugs will be used less in all health conditions including depression. Thomas Edison stated, "The doctor of the future will give no medicine, but will interest his patient in the care of the human frame, in diet and in the cause and prevention of disease." Edison's prophecy is destined to come true because it is so logical.

As medical understanding evolves, new paradigms develop. A paradigm refers to a model used to explain events. It is becoming more obvious that a new paradigm is emerging in medicine. While the old paradigm viewed the body basically as a machine, the new paradigm focuses on the interconnectedness of body, mind, emotions, social factors, and the environment in determining the status of health. Rather than relying on drugs and surgery, the new model utilizes natural, noninvasive techniques to promote health and healing.

It is my hope that the natural healing methods and techniques given in this book can be utilized by you or someone close to you in the achievement of greater health and happiness.

MICHAEL T. MURRAY, N.D.

Before you read on:

• Do not self-diagnose. Proper medical care is critical to good health. If you have symptoms suggestive of an illness discussed in this book, please consult a physician, preferably a naturopath (N.D.), holistic M.D. or D.O., chiropractor, or other natural health care specialist.

• If you are currently on a prescription medication such as Prozac, you absolutely must work with your doctor before discontinuing any drug. Discontinuing a prescription without medical supervision can be life-threatening.

• If you wish to try the natural approach, discuss it with your physician. Since your physician is most likely unaware of the natural alternatives available, you may need to educate him or her. Bring this book along with you to the doctor's office. The natural alternatives being recommended are based upon published studies in medical journals. Key references are provided if your physician wants additional information.

• Remember, although many natural alternatives, such as nutritional supplements and herbs, are effective on their own, they work even better if they are part of a comprehensive natural-treatment plan that focuses on diet and lifestyle factors. Do not underestimate the value of diet and lifestyle.

Contents

Contents

Natural Alternatives
to Prozac

Chapter 1

The Prozac Phenomenon

Hailed as a medical miracle by many and a dangerous psychoactive drug by others, Prozac is perhaps the most controversial drug ever marketed. Developed by Eli Lilly and Company, Prozac was launched in the United States in 1987 after fifteen years of clinical research. It has quickly become the most widely prescribed (and most profitable) antidepressant drug. Despite the tremendous publicity, Prozac is not a panacea for depression. In fact, it is no more effective than other antidepressants, including drugs that have been around since the 1950s. Prozac may not be more effective, but it is more expensive. The monthly cost for Prozac can range between $50 and $200 depending upon dosage while by comparison the monthly cost is around $7 for a generic tricyclic antidepressant. Detailed clinical studies indicate that roughly one third of patients with depression will either not be helped by Prozac and other anti-depressant drugs or will be unable to tolerate its side effects.

Why is Prozac so popular? The media has played a major role by publishing articles labeling Prozac as a major breakthrough in the treatment of depression. The public, hungry for information on this miracle "happy pill," kept psychiatrist Peter Kramer's pro-Prozac book, Listening to Prozac, on the New York Times best-seller list for nearly four months. In Kramer's book he advocated the use of Prozac for "cosmetic psychopharmacology" or as a "personality pill" in helping a normal person develop a more "socially rewarding personality." According to Dr. Kramer, "Prozac seems to fire confidence to the habitually timid, to make the sensitive brash, to lend the introvert the social skills of a salesman." Of course Dr. Kramer also points out that not all patients respond this way.

Another reason for its widespread popularity is that Prozac, as well as other antidepressant drugs, fits nicely into the dominant theoretical model of depression—the "biogenic amine" hypothesis. This model focuses more on biochemical factors in the brain causing depression rather than psychological factors. Perhaps the main reason this model is so popular is that it is a better fit for drug therapy. According to the biogenic amine hypothesis, depression is due to a biochemical deficiency characterized by imbalances of amino acids, which form neurotransmitters known as monoamines. Monoamines include serotonin, melatonin, dopamine, and norepinephrine. Environmental, nutritional, psychological, and genetic factors can all lead to an imbalance in the monoamines, which might result in depression. Monoamine neurotransmitters are released by brain cells to carry a chemical message by binding to receptor sites on neighboring brain cells. Almost as soon as the monoamine is released, enzymes are at work that will either breakdown the monoamine or work to uptake the monoamine back into the brain cell. Different antidepressant drugs act by increasing different monoamines in the brain by blocking either the re-uptake or the breakdown or by enhancing the effect of a specific monoamine.

It is interesting to note that the monoamines are manufactured from dietary amino acids, the building block molecules of proteins. For example, the amino acid tryptophan serves as the precursor to serotonin and melatonin, while phenylalanine and tyrosine are precursors to dopamine, epinephrine, and norepinephrine. These amino acids have proven to be effective natural antidepressants and are discussed in chapter 9.

How Does Prozac Work?

Prozac works by specifically inhibiting the re-uptake of serotonin at the nerve endings in the brain. As a result more serotonin is likely to bind to receptor sites on brain cells and transmit the serotonin signal. Serotonin is a very important neurotransmitter. It is the brain's own natural antidepressant and tranquilizer. A decrease in serotonin function is thought to be a major cause of depression, anxiety, and insomnia.[1]

Prozac and several other drugs (e.g., Effexor, Paxil, and Zoloft) are technically classified as a "selective serotonin re-uptake inhibitor" (SSRI). Other antidepressant drugs are classified according to their chemical structure and/or mechanism of action. Tricyclic drugs such as amitriptyline (Elavil, Endep) are also thought to inhibit the re-uptake of serotonin, but they are less selective than the newer drugs in that they also inhibit the re-uptake of norepinephrine. Monoamine oxidase inhibitors, such as phenelzine (Nardil) and tranylcypromine (Parnate), inhibit an enzyme (MAO type A) responsible for the breakdown of all monoamines; as a result levels of all monoamines are increased. Two other drugs, bupropion (Wellbutrin) and trazodone (Desyrel), are classified as miscellaneous antidepressants, although trazodone has exhibited selective serotonin re-uptake inhibition, and bupropion has been shown to inhibit the re-uptake of both serotonin and epinephrine.

Prozac and other antidepressants typically require at least a two-week period before any effects are observed.

Table 1.1 The Major Categories of Antidepressant Drugs

Serotonin re-uptake inhibitors	Tricyclic
fluoxetine (Prozac)	amitriptyline (Elavil, Endep)
venlafaxine (Effexor)	desipramine (Norpramin,
paroxetine (Paxil)	Pertofrane)
sertraline (Zoloft)	doxepin (Adapin, Sinequan)

Tricyclic (*cont.*)

imipramine (Imavate, Presa-
mine, Trofinil)

nortryptaline (Aventyl,
Pamelor)

protryptaline (Vivactil)

Tetracyclic

maprotiline (Ludiomil)

Monoamine oxidase inhibitors

phenelzine (Nardil)

tranylcypromine (Parnate)

Miscellaneous

bupropion (Wellbutrin)

trazodone (Desyrel)

Side Effects of Prozac and Other Antidepressant Drugs

While antidepressant drugs are successful in alleviating depression in many cases (60% to 75%), they are also associated with many side effects. Prozac is generally regarded as being better tolerated largely based on the fact that only 17% of patients taking Prozac discontinue treatment because of side effects compared with 31% of patients taking a tricyclic antidepressant. It should be clear that Prozac is regarded as being better tolerated only because side effects are so common with the other antidepressant drugs. Prozac is far from being classified as a well-tolerated drug, as results from clinical trials have demonstrated that 21% of patients taking the drug experience nausea; 20% headaches; 15% anxiety and nervousness; 14% insomnia; 12% drowsiness; 12% diarrhea; 9.5% dry mouth; 9% loss of appetite; 8% sweating and tremor; and 3% rash.[2] Prozac and other antidepressants inhibit sexual function. In studies where sexual side effects were thoroughly evaluated, 43% of men and women taking various antidepressants and 34% taking Prozac reported loss of libido or diminished sexual response.[3] The latest edition of the *Physician's Desk Reference* lists only 2% of patients suffer from sexual problems as a result of Prozac. This discrepancy is substantial and probably reflects difficulty in feeling comfortable talking about a sensitive subject by patients. The 43% level is probably more reflective of the degree of sexual problems caused by Prozac.

Prozac is more likely than other antidepressants to cause a condition called akathisia—a drug-induced state of agitation—and in some people, it may induce violent and destructive outbursts. The violent and suicidal reactions experienced by some patients taking Prozac have become so common and publicized that several citizens groups have formed to create awareness of these dangers of the drug. Although several studies have not shown an association between Prozac and suicide, these studies are offset by numerous case reports suggesting a strong link.[4] This controversy is discussed in greater detail below.

Benzodiazepines

Perhaps the only drug that rivals Prozac in terms of controversy is Valium, the widely used tranquilizer of the 1970s. Valium is a member of a group of drugs known as benzodiazepines. These drugs are primarily used for anxiety and insomnia. However, many physicians (particularly primary-care physicians) also prescribe benzodiazepines in the treatment of depression either alone or in combination with Prozac. Benzodiazepines act to enhance the action of the neurotransmitter gamma-aminobutyric acid (GABA), which in turn blocks the arousal of certain areas of the brain. Benzodiazepines are not designed to be used long-term, as they are addictive, associated with numerous side effects, and cause abnormal sleep patterns. They include the following:

alprazolam (*Xanax*)
chloazepate (*Tranxene*)
chlordiazepoxide (*Librium*)
clonazepam (*Klonopin*)
diazepam (*Valium*)
flurazepam (*Dalmane*)
lorazepam (*Ativan*)
halazepam (*Paxipam*)
oxazepam (*Serax*)
prazepam (*Centrax*)
tamazepam (*Restoril*)
triazolam (*Halcion*)

The benzodiazepines can produce many side effects. Because the drugs can produce dizziness, drowsiness, and impaired coordination, it is important not to drive or engage in any potentially dangerous activities while on these drugs. Alcohol should never be consumed with benzodiazepines.

Benzodiazepines will often produce a morning "hangover" feeling. Other possible side effects include allergic reactions, headache, blurred vision, nausea, indigestion, diarrhea or constipation, and lethargy.

The most serious side effects of the benzodiazepines relate to memory and behavior. Because the drugs act on brain chemistry, significant changes in brain function and behavior can occur. This can manifest as severe memory impairment and amnesia of events while on the drug, nervousness, confusion, hallucinations, bizarre behavior, and extreme irritability and aggressiveness. Benzodiazepines have also been shown to increase feelings of depression, including suicidal thinking.

Benzodiazepines, especially Halcion, have been receiving a great deal of negative attention in the media the past few years. More people are waking up to the fact that these drugs can be quite dangerous if used for other than occasional use. If you have taken a benzodiazepine for more than four weeks, do not stop taking the drug suddenly. It is important to work with your physician to taper off the drug gradually in order to avoid potentially dangerous withdrawal symptoms. Symptoms of withdrawal can include anxiety, irritability, sensations of panic, insomnia, nausea, headache, impaired concentration, memory loss, depression, extreme sensitivity to the environment, seizures, hallucinations, and paranoia.

The Dark Side of Prozac

Prozac has been one of the most controversial drugs ever developed because of its dark side, namely, its ability to cause violent, aggressive, and even suicidal behavior in some people.[5] The Citizen's Commission on Human Rights (an organization that is part of the Church of Scientology) obtained, through the Freedom of Information Act, the adverse drug-reaction reports on all of the major antidepressant drugs from 1985. During that time Prozac received 23,067 claims of adverse drug reactions (ADRs) compared with Elavil, a commonly used standby antidepressant, which received only 2,032. Suicide attempts in the Elavil group were 10, compared with 1,436 attempts with Prozac, and death rates in the Prozac group were 1,313 compared with 159 for Elavil. Of course Prozac's being the more prescribed of these two drugs helps explain this increase. But there does seem to be a problem with Prozac in some people.

Because of the negative publicity, the Food and Drug Administration (FDA) convened a special committee to examine the growing concern with Prozac. This committee included ten psychiatrists, and according to a lengthy and insightful report titled "Prozac, Eli Lilly and the FDA," which appeared in the *Townsend Letter for Doctors* in February 1993, Gary Null points out that when Dr. Martin Teicher, a Harvard researcher at the FDA hearing, began to present evidence of the possible link between Prozac and violent, suicidal thoughts, the panel refused to allow him to present his slides because they were not interested in his findings. Instead they allowed three slide presentations in defense of Prozac.[6]

The panel was not interested in some of the other points brought up by Dr. Teicher after he sat through the Eli Lilly–sponsored presentations. For example, in the presentation given by Jan Fawcett, a psychiatrist sponsored by Eli Lilly, it was pointed out that the common risk factors associated with suicide are anxiety, insomnia, panic attacks, and poor concentration. Dr. Teicher then stated that Eli Lilly's prescribing information for Prozac lists anxiety and insomnia as one of the most common side effects (see above), and if anxiety and insomnia are risk factors for suicide, isn't it safe to assume that there may be a link between Prozac and suicide? The FDA panel simply ignored Dr. Teicher when he pointed out the contradiction.

According to Mr. Null's report, the FDA panel received enough evidence linking Prozac and violent behavior to take action against the drug, but for some reason they chose not to. Mr. Null felt conflict of interest may have been the reason. Nine of the ten members of the panel had financial conflicts of interest, for example, Jeffrey Lieberman, a psychiatrist, who at the time he sat on the panel had received $20,000 in grants from Sandoz, the manufacturer of Pamelor, the second most widely prescribed antidepressant.

Psychiatrist James Claghorn received $170,000 worth of grants from makers of antidepressants. It is interesting to note that Dr. Claghorn gave positive reviews of two other antidepressant drugs in the 1980s—zimelidine and nomifensine.

Within two years of his review both drugs were pulled off the market due to serious side effects.

Psychiatrist David Dunner had financial compensation of over a half a million dollars from four manufacturers of antidepressants. Remarkably, Dr. Dunner even had $200,000 worth of grants "pending" from Eli Lilly, Prozac's maker, when the hearing took place. Upon review of Dr. Dunner's conflict-of-interest waiver the Citizen's Commission on Human Rights discovered his did not include several relevant items. The conflicts not disclosed in Dr. Dunner's waiver included the following: two pending grants worth $250,000 from antidepressant drug makers and an engagement to speak at a series of seminars funded by Eli Lilly. Dr. Dunner failed to mention these conflicts. In fact in his waiver Dr. Dunner stated that he had no current commitments to speak.

These omissions may have slipped Dr. Dunner's mind. But even without them he certainly should have not been on the panel. After all, here was a situation where a psychiatrist had received over $4 million worth of research grants from antidepressant manufacturers in an eight-year period prior to the FDA hearings to discuss taking these very same drugs off the market.

It must also be pointed out that according to Peter Breggin, M.D., coauthor of *Talking Back to Prozac* (St. Martin's Press, 1993), the studies the FDA used to approve Prozac were unconvincing. Dr. Breggin first points out that contrary to widespread belief, the FDA does not conduct any of the studies used for drug approval; the studies are financed, constructed, and supervised by drug companies using doctors and researchers they hire. He then goes on to detail how many of the clinical studies were flawed. Because most of the studies were flawed, the FDA found only four studies worthy enough to consider. One of these showed Prozac to be no better than a placebo. Three others supposedly showed Prozac to be more effective than the placebo, but not as good as older antidepressants. Clouding the results of these studies was a high dropout rate due to lack of effectiveness and side effects. Although Prozac has been studied in over 11,000 patients, only 286 patients completed the four- to six-week trials the FDA used to approve Prozac.

Dr. Breggin believes Prozac's true effect is that it acts as a stimulant similar to amphetamines. There are many similarities between the two classes of drugs. Both are capable of inducing nervousness, anxiety, insomnia, agitation, and loss of appetite, as well as behavioral abnormalities such as paranoia, violence, and suicide. Dr. Breggin does not believe Prozac has any real antidepressant effect.

Perhaps the most alarming thing to realize with Prozac is that there have been no long-term studies. People taking Prozac are the equivalent of human guinea pigs. Prozac has been shown to cause cancer in experimental studies.[7] Dr. Lorne Brandes of the Manitoba Institute of Cell Biology in Winnipeg, has conducted detailed studies in animals that demonstrate that when Prozac (as well as other antidepressants) was given at doses comparable to those given to humans, tumor growth and the number of tumors was significantly greater than control animals not given Prozac.

These results raise many questions concerning the safety of Prozac. Dr. Brandes's results call into question the use of Prozac and other antidepressants.

Final Comments

The majority of patients on Prozac are women between the ages of twenty-five and fifty. The overwhelming majority of the nearly one million prescriptions being written for Prozac each month are not by psychiatrists, but rather by primary-care doctors and non–mental health specialists.[8] Hopefully, but not always, when psychiatrists prescribe Prozac, they consider drug education and psychotherapy. However, psychotherapy (nondrug therapy) accounts for only about 8 percent of dollars spent on mental health. The majority of the money is being spent on office calls for the prescribing and monitoring of drugs.[9] When primary-care doctors and non–mental health specialists prescribe Prozac, drug education and psychotherapy are even more rare, since the average primary-care physician spends three minutes or less with his or her depressed patients.[10]

Obviously there must be a better approach to depression than simply prescribing a drug like Prozac. Such an approach is described in the following chapters.

Chapter 2

A Different View
of Depression

Modern psychiatry focuses on correcting the chemical changes in the neurotransmitters of the brain that produce depression rather than identifying and eliminating the psychological factors that are responsible for producing the imbalances in serotonin, dopamine, GABA, and other neurotransmitters. This chapter presents a different model of depression—the learned helplessness model—and provides recommendations for dealing with depression by creating a more optimistic outlook. However, let us first define depression.

Depression Defined

Clinical depression is more than feeling depressed. The official definition of clinical depression, as defined by the American Psychiatric Association in its *Diagnostic and Statistical Manual of Mental Disorders (DSM-IV)*, is based upon the following eight primary criteria:

- Poor appetite with weight loss, or increased appetite with weight gain
- Insomnia or hypersomnia (wanting to sleep all of the time)
- Physical hyperactivity or inactivity
- Loss of interest or pleasure in usual activities, or decrease in sexual drive
- Loss of energy and feelings of fatigue
- Feelings of worthlessness, self-reproach, or inappropriate guilt
- Diminished ability to think or concentrate
- Recurrent thoughts of death or suicide

The presence of five of these eight symptoms definitely indicates clinical depression; the individual with four is probably depressed. According to the *DSM-IV*, the depressed state must be present for at least one month to be called depression. Clinical depression is also referred to as major depression or unipolar depression.

Dysthymia

Obviously, there is a spectrum of clinical depression that ranges from mild feelings of depression to serious considerations of suicide. Mild depression is also known as dysthymia. *Dysthymia* is a term coined in the 1980s and replaced the term *depressive neurosis* that was used in the 1950s and the term *depressive personality* that was used in the 1970s. Like clinical depression, dysthymia is diagnosed according to *DSM-IV* criteria. In order to be officially diagnosed as dysthymic, a patient must be depressed most of the time for at least two years (one year for children or adolescents) and have at least three of the following symptoms:

- Low self-esteem or lack of self-confidence
- Pessimism, hopelessness, or despair
- Lack of interest in ordinary pleasures and activities
- Withdrawal from social activities
- Fatigue or lethargy
- Guilt or ruminating about the past
- Irritability or excessive anger
- Lessened productivity
- Difficulty concentrating or making decisions

Bipolar (Manic) Depression and Hypomania

Bipolar depression is a disorder characterized by periods of major depression alternating with periods of elevated mood. If the elevated mood is relatively mild and lasts for four days or less, it is referred to as hypomania. Mania is longer and more intense. To be diagnosed as a bipolar depressive, an individual would be expected to have at least three of the following symptoms:

- Excessive self-esteem or grandiosity
- Reduced need for sleep
- Extreme talkativeness, excessive telephoning
- Extremely rapid flight of thoughts along with the feeling that the mind is racing
- Inability to concentrate, easily distracted
- Increase in social or work-oriented activities, often with a sixty- to eighty-hour work week
- Poor judgment, as indicated by sprees of uncontrolled spending, increased sexual indiscretions, and misguided financial decisions

A full-blown manic attack requires hospitalization. Manic people have lost control; they may hurt themselves or others. The standard treatment for bipolar depression is lithium. Lithium stabilizes mood. It is especially useful in preventing the manic phase. Lithium is used either alone or in combination with an antidepressant such as Prozac. However, because Prozac and other antidepressant drugs can occasionally induce mania and hypomania, it is often very difficult to deal effectively with the lows in bipolar depressives with drug therapy.

Seasonal Affective Disorder

Another form of depression is known as seasonal affective disorder (SAD). Individuals diagnosed as suffering from SAD experience regularly occurring winter depression. Typically these individuals feel depressed, slow down, and generally oversleep, overeat, and crave carbohydrates in the winter. In the summer these same patients feel elated, active, and energetic. Although many variables may be responsible for SAD, light exposure appears the most logical explanation. It is well known that other mammals exhibit seasonal variation in activities, sleep patterns, and appetite and are extremely sensitive to changes in day length. The key hormonal change may be a reduced secretion of melatonin from the pineal gland and an increased secretion of cortisol by the adrenal glands. Melatonin supplementation may improve SAD because it not only increases brain melatonin levels but also may suppress cortisol secretion.[1] Melatonin is discussed in Chapter 10.

Another natural therapy that has shown impressive results is full-spectrum light therapy. The antidepressive effects of full-spectrum light therapy have been demonstrated in well-monitored, controlled studies, not only in SAD but also in clinical depression.[2] It is thought that the antidepressant effect of light therapy is probably due to its ability to restore proper melatonin synthesis and secretion by the pineal gland leading to reestablishment of the proper circadian rhythm—the internal clock that signals the secretion of various hormones at different times to regulate body functions.

Light therapy consists of using full-spectrum lighting (Vitalite is a popular brand). The typical protocol used in clinical studies involves placing full-spectrum fluorescent tubes in a regular fluorescent fixture (eight tubes total). Patients are then instructed to sit three feet away from the light from 5:00 A.M. to 8:00 A.M. and again from 5:30 P.M. to 8:30 P.M. They are free to engage in activities as long as they glance at the light at least once per minute. Obviously to adopt this treatment protocol would greatly restrict social activities. Something that may work just as well is simply replacing standard light bulbs with full-spectrum light bulbs.

Another natural treatment that has been shown to improve SAD is the St. John's wort extract standardized to contain 0.3% hypericin (discussed in Chapter 6) at a dosage of 300 mg three times daily.[3]

Test Your Depression

A widely used test for determining depression is the CES-D (Center for Epidemiological Studies–Depression) developed by Lenore Radloff at the National Institute for Mental Health. This depression self-test does not diagnose clinical depression, but it can be used to determine your relative level of depression. Simply circle the best description of how you have felt over the past week:

1. I was bothered by things that usually don't bother me.

    0   Rarely or none of the time (less than 1 day)
    1   Some or a little of the time (1–2 days)
    2   Occasionally or a moderate amount of the time (3–4 days)
    3   Most or all of the time (5–7 days)

2. I did not feel like eating; my appetite was poor.

    0   Rarely or none of the time (less than 1 day)
    1   Some or a little of the time (1–2 days)
    2   Occasionally or a moderate amount of the time (3–4 days)
    3   Most or all of the time (5–7 days)

3. I felt that I could not shake off the blues even with help from my family and friends.

    0   Rarely or none of the time (less than 1 day)
    1   Some or a little of the time (1–2 days)
    2   Occasionally or a moderate amount of the time (3–4 days)
    3   Most or all of the time (5–7 days)

4. I felt that I was not as good as other people.

    0   Rarely or none of the time (less than 1 day)
    1   Some or a little of the time (1–2 days)
    2   Occasionally or a moderate amount of the time (3–4 days)
    3   Most or all of the time (5–7 days)

5. I had trouble keeping my mind on what I was doing.

    0   Rarely or none of the time (less than 1 day)
    1   Some or a little of the time (1–2 days)
    2   Occasionally or a moderate amount of the time (3–4 days)
    3   Most or all of the time (5–7 days)

6. I felt depressed.

    0   Rarely or none of the time (less than 1 day)
    1   Some or a little of the time (1–2 days)
    2   Occasionally or a moderate amount of the time (3–4 days)
    3   Most or all of the time (5–7 days)

7. I felt that everything I did was an effort.

    0   Rarely or none of the time (less than 1 day)
    1   Some or a little of the time (1–2 days)
    2   Occasionally or a moderate amount of the time (3–4 days)
    3   Most or all of the time (5–7 days)

8. I felt hopeless about the future.

   0 Rarely or none of the time (less than 1 day)
   1 Some or a little of the time (1–2 days)
   2 Occasionally or a moderate amount of the time (3–4 days)
   3 Most or all of the time (5–7 days)

9. I thought my life had been a failure.

   0 Rarely or none of the time (less than 1 day)
   1 Some or a little of the time (1–2 days)
   2 Occasionally or a moderate amount of the time (3–4 days)
   3 Most or all of the time (5–7 days)

10. I felt fearful.

   0 Rarely or none of the time (less than 1 day)
   1 Some or a little of the time (1–2 days)
   2 Occasionally or a moderate amount of the time (3–4 days)
   3 Most or all of the time (5–7 days)

11. My sleep was restless.

   0 Rarely or none of the time (less than 1 day)
   1 Some or a little of the time (1–2 days)
   2 Occasionally or a moderate amount of the time (3–4 days)
   3 Most or all of the time (5–7 days)

12. I was unhappy.

    0   Rarely or none of the time (less than 1 day)
    1   Some or a little of the time (1–2 days)
    2   Occasionally or a moderate amount of the time (3–4 days)
    3   Most or all of the time (5–7 days)

13. I talked less than usual.

    0   Rarely or none of the time (less than 1 day)
    1   Some or a little of the time (1–2 days)
    2   Occasionally or a moderate amount of the time (3–4 days)
    3   Most or all of the time (5–7 days)

14. I felt lonely.

    0   Rarely or none of the time (less than 1 day)
    1   Some or a little of the time (1–2 days)
    2   Occasionally or a moderate amount of the time (3–4 days)
    3   Most or all of the time (5–7 days)

15. People were unfriendly.

    0   Rarely or none of the time (less than 1 day)
    1   Some or a little of the time (1–2 days)
    2   Occasionally or a moderate amount of the time (3–4 days)
    3   Most or all of the time (5–7 days)

16. I did not enjoy life.

    0   Rarely or none of the time (less than 1 day)
    1   Some or a little of the time (1–2 days)
    2   Occasionally or a moderate amount of the time (3–4 days)
    3   Most or all of the time (5–7 days)

17. I had crying spells.

    0   Rarely or none of the time (less than 1 day)
    1   Some or a little of the time (1–2 days)
    2   Occasionally or a moderate amount of the time (3–4 days)
    3   Most or all of the time (5–7 days)

18. I felt sad.

    0   Rarely or none of the time (less than 1 day)
    1   Some or a little of the time (1–2 days)
    2   Occasionally or a moderate amount of the time (3–4 days)
    3   Most or all of the time (5–7 days)

19. I felt that people disliked me.

    0   Rarely or none of the time (less than 1 day)
    1   Some or a little of the time (1–2 days)
    2   Occasionally or a moderate amount of the time (3–4 days)
    3   Most or all of the time (5–7 days)

20. I could not get "going."

   0   Rarely or none of the time (less than 1 day)
   1   Some or a little of the time (1–2 days)
   2   Occasionally or a moderate amount of the time (3–4 days)
   3   Most or all of the time (5–7 days)

To score your test, simply add up all the numbers that you circled. If your score was from 0 to 9, congratulations! If your score was 10 to 15, you may be mildly depressed. A score between 16 and 24 indicates that depression may be more of a problem for you. If your score was over 24, you are most likely very depressed. Regardless of your score, you will find the rest of this chapter fascinating and beneficial in lowering your degree of depression.

The Learned Helplessness Model

Although the biogenic amine model of depression is the dominant medical model of depression, there are several other models, based on social and psychological factors. The one that I feel has the most merit is the learned helplessness model developed by Martin Seligman, Ph.D. I believe that Dr. Seligman's contributions to the understanding of human behavior are on a par with Albert Einstein's contributions to physics and Linus Pauling's contributions to biochemistry. Much of what will be presented in the rest of this chapter is based upon Dr. Seligman's work. If you are interested in learning more about this incredible scientist, I encourage you to read his books, *Learned Optimism* (Knopf, 1991) and *What You Can Change & What You Can't* (Knopf, 1993).

One of Dr. Seligman's major contributions to psychology was the development of an animal model known as the learned helplessness model of depression. During the 1960s Dr. Seligman discovered that animals could be trained to be helpless. Let me describe one of his classic experiments.

The experiment was performed on three groups of dogs. The first group of dogs was given an escapable electrical shock. The dogs could turn off the shock by simply pressing a panel with their noses. This group of dogs would thus have control. The second group of dogs was "yoked" to the first group. They would get exactly the same shocks as the first group but would be unable to turn off the shock. The shock would cease only when the "yoked" dog in the first group would press its nose to the panel. Thus, the second group had no control over the degree of shock they received. The third group of dogs would get no shocks at all.

Once the dogs went through this first part of the experiment, they would be placed in what is known as a shuttle box—a box separated in the middle by a small barrier that the dogs could jump over. The dogs would be electrically shocked, but they would be able to escape the shock by simply jumping over the barrier to the other side. Dr. Seligman believed that the first and third groups would quickly figure this out, but he felt the second group of dogs would have learned to be helpless in that they would believe that nothing they could do would matter. Dr. Seligman thought that the dogs in the second group would simply lie down and accept the shock.

Here were the results: The first and third groups of dogs learned within seconds that they could avoid the shock by jumping over the barrier. In contrast, the dogs in the second group would simply lie down and not even make an effort to jump over the barrier, even though they could see the shockless side of the shuttle box.

You might think that this experiment applies only to dogs, rats, and other animals and that humans, because of higher cognitive functions, would never react in a similar fashion. But Dr. Seligman and his colleagues went on to show that many humans react in an identical fashion to animals in these experiments.

What significance do these experiments have for depression? Seligman's learned helplessness model became an effective experiment to test antidepressive drugs. Basically, when animals that had learned to be helpless were given antidepressant drugs, they would unlearn helplessness and start exerting control over their environment. Scientists discovered that when animals learned to be helpless, it resulted in alteration of brain monoamine content. The drugs would restore proper monoamine balance and alter the animal's behavior. Researchers would also learn that when animals with learned helplessness were taught how to gain control over their environment, brain chemistry also normalized.

The alteration in brain monoamine content in the animals with learned helplessness mirrors the altered monoamine content in human depression. What all the research indicates is that learned helplessness in animals and depression in humans can be improved either by antidepressant drugs or through retraining.

While most physicians quickly look to drugs to alter brain chemistry, helping the patient gain greater control over his or her life will actually produce even greater biochemical changes. One of the most powerful techniques to produce the necessary biochemical changes in the brains of depressed individuals is teaching them to be more optimistic.

Outside the laboratory setting, Dr. Seligman discovered that the determining factor on how a person would react to uncontrollable events, either "bad" or "good," was his explanatory style—the way in which he explained events. Optimistic people were immune to becoming helpless and depressed. However, individuals that were pessimistic were extremely likely to become depressed when something went wrong in their lives. Dr. Seligman and other researchers also found a direct correlation between an individual's level of optimism and the likeliness of developing not only clinical depression but other illnesses as well.[4] In one of the longer studies, patients were followed for a total of thirty-five years. While optimists rarely got depressed, pessimists were extremely likely to battle depression and other psychological disturbances.

Test Your Optimism

Now is a good time to test your optimism. We will use a simple test Dr. Seligman developed—the Seligman Attributional Style Questionnaire. Take as much time as you need to answer each of the questions. There are no right or wrong answers. It is important that you take the test before you read the interpretation. Read the description of each situation and vividly imagine it happening to you. Choose the response that most applies to you by circling either A or B. Ignore the letter and number codes for now; they will be explained latter.

1. The project you are in charge of is a great success.

    PsG

    A. I kept a close watch over everyone's work.   1
    B. Everyone devoted a lot of time and energy
       to it.   0

2. You and your spouse (boyfriend/girlfriend) make up after a fight.

    PmG

    A. I forgave him/her.   0
    B. I'm usually forgiving.   1

3. You get lost driving to a friend's house.

	PsB
A. I missed a turn.	1
B. My friend gave me bad directions.	0

4. Your spouse (boyfriend/girlfriend) surprises you with a gift.

	PsG
A. He/she just got a raise at work.	0
B. I took him/her out to a special dinner the night before.	1

5. You forget your spouse's (boyfriend's/girlfriend's) birthday.

	PmB
A. I'm not good at remembering birthdays.	1
B. I was preoccupied with other things.	0

6. You get a flower from a secret admirer.

	PvG
A. I am attractive to him/her.	0
B. I am a popular person.	1

7. You run for a community office position and you win.

	PvG
A. I devote a lot of time and energy to campaigning.	0
B. I work very hard at everything I do.	1

8. You miss an important engagement.

                                                        PvB

    A. Sometimes my memory fails me.   1

    B. I sometimes forget to check my appointment
book.   0

9. You run for a community office position and you lose.

                                                          PsB

    A. I didn't campaign hard enough.   1

    B. The person who won knew more people.   0

10. You host a successful dinner.

                                                       PmG

    A. I was particularly charming that night. 0

    B. I am a good host.   1

11. You stop a crime by calling the police.

                                                          PsG

    A. A strange noise caught my attention.   0

    B. I was alert that day.   1

12. You were extremely healthy all year.

                                                            PsG

    A. Few people around me were sick, so I wasn't
exposed.   0

    B. I made sure I ate well and got enough rest. 1

13. You owe the library ten dollars for an overdue book.

	PmB
A. When I am really involved in what I am reading, I often forget when it's due.	1
B. I was so involved in writing the report that I forgot to return the book.	0

14. Your stocks make you a lot of money.

	PmG
A. My broker decided to take on something new.	0
B. My broker is a top-notch investor.	1

15. You win an athletic contest.

	PmG
A. I was feeling unbeatable.	0
B. I train hard.	1

16. You fail an important examination.

	PsB
A. I wasn't as smart as the other people taking the exam.	1
B. I didn't prepare for it well.	0

17. You prepared a special meal for a friend and he/she barely touched the food.

	PvB
A. I wasn't a good cook.	1
B. I made the meal in a rush.	0

18. You lose a sporting event for which you have been train-ing for a long time.

	PvB
A. I'm not very athletic.	1
B. I'm not good at that sport.	0

19. Your car runs out of gas on a dark street late at night.

	PsB
A. I didn't check to see how much gas was in the tank.	1
B. The gas gauge was broken.	0

20. You lose your temper with a friend.

	PmB
A. He/she is always nagging me.	1
B. He/she was in a hostile mood.	0

21. You are penalized for not returning your income tax forms on time.

	PmB
A. I always put off doing my taxes.	1
B. I was lazy about getting my taxes done this year.	0

22. You ask a person out on a date and he/she says no.

	PvB
A. I was a wreck that day.	1
B. I got tongue-tied when I asked him/her on the date.	0

23. A game show host picks you out of the audience to participate in the show.

	PsG
A. I was sitting in the right seat.	0
B. I looked the most enthusiastic.	1

24. You are frequently asked to dance at a party.

	PmG
A. I am outgoing at parties.	1
B. I was in perfect form that night.	0

25. You buy your spouse (boyfriend/girlfriend) a gift and he/she doesn't like it.

	PsB
A. I don't put enough thought into things like that.	1
B. He/she has very picky tastes.	0

26. You do exceptionally well in a job interview.

        PmG

    A. I felt extremely confident during the interview.   0
    B. I interview well.   1

27. You tell a joke and everyone laughs.

        PsG

    A. The joke was funny.   0
    B. My timing was perfect.   1

28. Your boss gives you too little time in which to finish a project, but you get it finished anyway.

        PvG

    A. I am good at my job.   0
    B. I am an efficient person.   1

29. You've been feeling run-down lately.

        PmB

    A. I never get a chance to relax.   1
    B. I was exceptionally busy this week.   0

30. You ask someone to dance and he/she says no.

        PsB

    A. I am not a good enough dancer.   1
    B. He/she doesn't like to dance.   0

31. You save a person from choking to death.

	PvG
A. I know a technique to stop someone from choking.	0
B. I know what to do in crisis situations.	1

32. Your romantic partner wants to cool things off for a while.

	PvB
A. I'm too self-centered.	1
B. I don't spend enough time with him/her.	0

33. A friend says something that hurts your feelings.

	PmB
A. She always blurts things out without thinking of others.	1
B. My friend was in a bad mood and took it out on me.	0

34. Your employer comes to you for advice.

	PvG
A. I am an expert in the area about which I was asked.	0
B. I'm good at giving useful advice.	1

35. A friend thanks you for helping him/her get through a bad time.

	PvG
A. I enjoy helping him/her through tough times.	0
B. I care about people.	1

36. You have a wonderful time at a party.

	PsG
A. Everyone was friendly.	0
B. I was friendly.	1

37. Your doctor tells you that you are in good physical shape.

	PvG
A. I make sure I exercise frequently.	0
B. I am very health-conscious.	1

38. Your spouse (boyfriend/girlfriend) takes you away for a romantic weekend.

	PmG
A. He/she needed to get away for a few days.	0
B. He/she likes to explore new areas.	1

39. Your doctor tells you that you eat too much sugar.

	PsB
A. I don't pay much attention to my diet.	1
B. You can't avoid sugar, it's in everything.	0

40. You are asked to head an important project.

	PmG
A. I just successfully completed a similar project.	0
B. I am a good supervisor.	1

41. You and your spouse (boyfriend/girlfriend) have been fighting a great deal.

	PsB
A. I have been feeling cranky and pressured lately.	1
B. He/she has been hostile lately.	0

42. You fall down a great deal while skiing.

	PmB
A. Skiing is difficult.	1
B. The trails were icy.	0

43. You win a prestigious award.

	PvG
A. I solved an important problem.	0
B. I was the best employee.	1

44. Your stocks are at an all-time low.

                                                    PvB

   A. I didn't know much about the business
      climate at the time.   1
   B. I made a poor choice of stocks.   0

45. You win the lottery.

                                                    PsG

   A. It was pure chance.   0
   B. I picked the right numbers.   1

46. You gain weight over the holidays and you can't lose it.

                                                    PmB

   A. Diets don't work in the long run.   1
   B. The diet I tried didn't work.   0

47. You are in the hospital and few people come to visit.

                                                    PsB

   A. I'm irritable when I am sick.   1
   B. My friends are negligent about things like
      that.   0

48. They won't honor your credit card at a store.

                                                    PvB

   A. I sometimes overestimate how much money
      I have.   1
   B. I sometimes forget to pay my credit card bill. 0

SCORING KEY

PmB ___	PmG ___
PvB ___	PvG ___
HoB ___	
PsB ___	PsG ___
Total B ___	Total G ___
G-B ___	

Interpreting Your Test

The test results will give you a clue as to your explanatory style. In other words the results will tell you about the way in which you explain things to yourself. It tells you your habit of thought. Again, remember there are no right or wrong answers.

There are three crucial dimensions to your explanatory style: permanence, pervasiveness, and personalization. Each dimension, plus a couple of others, will be scored from your test.

PERMANENCE

When pessimists are faced with challenges or bad events, they view these events as being permanent. By contrast people who are optimists tend to view the challenges or bad events as temporary. Here are some statements that reflect some subtle differences:

Permanent (Pessimistic):

"My boss is always a jerk."

"You never listen."

"This bad luck will never stop."

Temporary (Optimistic):

"My boss is in a bad mood to-day."

"You are not listening."

"My luck has got to turn."

To determine how you view bad events, look at the eight items coded PmB (for Permanent Bad): 5, 13, 20, 21, 29, 33, 42, and 46. Each one with 0 after it is optimistic, each one followed by a 1 is pessimistic. Total the numbers at the right-hand margin of the questions coded PmB and write the total on the PmB line on the scoring key.

If you totaled 0 or 1, you are very optimistic on this dimension; 2 or 3 is a moderately optimistic score; 4 is average; 5 or 6 is quite pessimistic; a 7 or 8 is extremely pessimistic.

Now let's take a look at the difference in explanatory style between pessimists and optimists when there is a positive event in their lives. It's just the opposite of what happened with a bad event. Pessimists view positive events as temporary, while optimists view them as permanent. Here again are some subtle differences in how pessimists and optimists might communicate their good fortune:

Temporary (Pessimistic)

"It's my lucky day."

"My opponent was off today."

"I tried hard today."

Permanent (Optimistic)

"I am always lucky."

"I am getting better everyday."

"I always give my best."

Now total all the questions coded PmG (for Permanent Good): 2, 10, 14, 15, 24, 26, 38, and 40. Write the total on the line in the scoring key marked PmG.

If you totaled 7 or 8, you are very optimistic on this dimension; 6 is a moderately optimistic score; 4 or 5 is average; 3 is pessimistic; a 0, 1 or 2 is extremely pessimistic.

Are you starting to see a pattern? If you are scoring as a pessimist, you may want to learn how to be more optimistic. Your anxiety may be due to your belief that bad things are always going to happen, while good things are only a fluke.

PERVASIVENESS

Pervasiveness describes the tendency to describe things either in universals (*everyone, always, never,* etc.) versus specifics (a specific individual, a specific time, etc.). Pessimists tend to describe things in universals, whereas optimists describe things in specifics.

Universal (Pessimists)	Specific (Optimist)
"All lawyers are jerks."	*"My attorney was a jerk."*
"Instruction manuals are worthless."	*"This instruction manual is worthless."*
"He is repulsive."	*"He is repulsive to me."*

Total your score for the questions coded PvB (for Pervasive Bad): 8, 17, 18, 22, 32, 44, and 48. Write the total on the PvB line.

If you totaled 0 or 1, you are very optimistic on this dimension; 2 or 3 is a moderately optimistic score; 4 is average; 5 or 6 is quite pessimistic; a 7 or 8 is extremely pessimistic.

Now let's look at the level of pervasiveness of good events. Optimists tend to view good events as universal, whereas pessimists view them as specific. Again, it's just the opposite of how each views a bad event.

Total your score for the questions coded PvG (for Pervasive Good): 6, 7, 28, 31, 34, 35, 37, and 43. And write the total on the line labeled PvG.

If you totaled 7 or 8, you are very optimistic on this dimension; 6 is a moderately optimistic score; 4 or 5 is average; 3 is pessimistic; a 0, 1, or 2 is extremely pessimistic.

HOPE

The level of hope or hopelessness is determined by our combined level of permanence and pervasiveness. Your level of hope may be the most significant score for this test. Take your PvB and add it to your PmB score. This is your hope score.

If it is 0, 1, or 2, you are extraordinarily hopeful; 3, 4, 5, or 6 is a moderately hopeful score; 7 or 8 is average; 9, 10, or 11 is moderately hopeless; and 12, 13, 14, 15, or 16 is severely hopeless.

People who make permanent and universal explanations for their troubles tend to suffer from stress, anxiety, and depression as well as collapse when things go bad. According to Dr. Seligman, no other score is as important as your hope score.

PERSONALIZATION

The final aspect of explanatory style is personalization. When bad things happen, we can either blame ourselves (internalize) and lower our self-esteem as a consequence or we can blame things beyond our control (externalize). Although it may not be right to deny personal responsibility, people who tend to externalize bad events have higher self-esteem and are more optimistic. Here are some examples:

Total your score for those questions coded PsB (for Personalization Bad): 3, 9, 16, 19, 25, 30, 39, 41, and 47.

A score of 0 or 1 indicates very high self-esteem and optimism; 2 or 3 indicates moderate self-esteem; 4 is average; 5 or 6 indicates moderately low self esteem; and 7 or 8 indicates very low self-esteem.

Now let's take a look at personalization and good events. Again, just the exact opposite occurs compared with bad events. When good things happen, the person with high self-esteem internalizes, while the person with low self-esteem externalizes.

Total your score for those questions coded PsG (for Personalization Good): 1, 4, 11, 12, 23, 27, 36, and 45. Write your score on the line marked PsG on your scoring key.

If you totaled 7 or 8, you are very optimistic on this dimension; 6 is a moderately optimistic score; 4 or 5 is average; 3 is pessimistic; a 0, 1, or 2 is extremely pessimistic.

YOUR OVERALL SCORES

To compute your overall scores, first add the three B's (PmB + PvB + PsB). This is your B (bad event) score. Do the same for all of the G's (PmG + PvG + PsG). This is your G (good event) score. Subtract B from G; this is your overall score.

If your B score is from 3 to 6, you are marvelously optimistic when bad events occur; 10 or 11 is average; 12 to 14 is pessimistic; anything above 14 is extremely pessimistic.

If your G score is 19 or above, you are extremely optimistic; 14 to 16 is average; 11 to 13 indicates pessimism; and a score of 10 or less indicates great pessimism.

If your overall score (G minus B) is above 8, you are very optimistic across the board; if it's from 6 to 8, you are moderately optimistic; 3 to 5 is average; 1 or 2 is pessimistic; and a score of zero or below is very pessimistic.

Learning Optimism

Optimists are healthier, happier, and enjoy life at a much higher level than pessimists. If that doesn't convince you to become an optimist, perhaps this will: Optimists earn over three times the income of pessimists.[5]

If you tend to battle depression, it is absolutely crucial that you become an optimistic person. Learning to be optimistic means that you have got to get in the habit of thinking with a positive attitude. If you are pessimistic, it is only because you have gotten into the habit of thinking in a negative framework.

Fortunately, Dr. Seligman believes that nature has equipped humans with an optimistic attitude. Optimism is what fuels human growth and development. The first step in building an optimistic or positive mental attitude is taking personal responsibility for your own positive mental state, your life, your current situation, and your health. The next step is taking action to make the changes you desire. Some of the natural antidepressants, especially St. John's wort extract, can be used as a crutch to improve your mood while your brain is being reprogrammed to be optimistic.

To help you become more optimistic, I am going to give you three valuable tips.

TIP I: BECOME A STUDENT OF OPTIMISM

One of the best ways to learn how to be more optimistic is to study optimism. The best way to become an expert in optimism is to read books that provide "blueprints" for optimism. In addition to Dr. Seligman's book *Learned Optimism,* here are a number of other books that I have found extremely helpful in my own life as well as in the lives of some of my patients:

The 7 Habits of Highly Effective People by Steven Covey (Simon and Schuster, 1989)

Bringing Out the Best in People by Alan Loy McGinnis (Augsberg, 1985)

Awaken the Giant Within by Anthony Robbins (Simon and Schuster, 1991)

Sound Mind, Sound Body by Dr. Kenneth R. Pelletier (Simon and Schuster, 1991)

See You at the Top by Zig Zigler (Pelican Publishing, 1975)

I also recommend that you listen to motivational and/or relaxation tapes on a regular basis. They are food for a positive attitude.

TIP 2: CONDITION YOUR MIND AND ATTITUDE

Our attitude is like our physical body, it needs conditioning to function properly. Conditioning the mind and attitude involves setting goals, paying attention to self-talk, creating and reciting affirmations, and asking empowering questions. Here are some exercises to perform for your attitude. You will need to get a notebook that you can write in. This notebook will become your personal success journal.

Exercise I—Goal Setting

Learning to set goals in a way that results in a positive experience is critical to achieving a positive attitude and high self-esteem. Here are four steps to setting goals:

1. State the goal in positive terms; do not use any negative words in your goal statement. For example it is better to say "I enjoy eating healthy, low-calorie, nutritious foods" than "I will not eat sugar, candy, ice cream, and other fat-

tening foods." Remember, always state the goal in positive terms and do not use any negative words in the goal statement.

2. Make your goal attainable and realistic. Again, goals can be used to create a success cycle and positive self-image. Little things add up to make a major difference in the way you feel about yourself. Each day write out a daily goal list, place even simple things on it that you want to accomplish during the day (e.g., "I will exercise for thirty minutes," "I will drink eight glasses of water," "I will take my vitamins," etc.) and check them off.

3. Be specific. The more clearly your goal is defined, the more likely you are to reach it. For example if you want to lose weight, what is the weight you desire? What is the body fat percentage or measurements you desire? Clearly define what it is you want to achieve.

4. State the goal in present tense, not future tense. In order to reach your goal, you have to believe you have already attained it. As noted psychologist Dr. Wayne Dyer says, "You'll see it, when you believe it." You must literally program yourself to achieve the goal. See and feel yourself having already achieved the goal, and success will be yours. Remember, always state your goal in the present tense.

Exercise 2—Positive Affirmations

An affirmation is a positive statement. Affirmations can make imprints on the subconscious mind to create a healthy, positive self-image. In addition affirmations can actually fuel the changes you desire. Like goals, affirmations must be phrased in the present tense and be stated in a positive way. Keep the affirmation short and simple but full of feeling. The more feeling that can be associated with the affirmation, the more powerful the impact on the subconscious mind. Visualize the affirmation; imagine yourself really experiencing what you are affirming.

Here are some examples of positive affirmations:

- I am a whole and complete person.
- I am in control of my life.
- I am an open channel of love and joy.
- I am filled with peace and wisdom.
- I am good to my body.
- I am growing stronger every day.

Using the above guidelines and examples, write down five affirmations that apply to you. State these affirmations aloud for a total of five minutes each day.

Exercise 3—Ask Empowering Questions

Our self-talk determines the quality of our lives. Especially the questions we habitually ask our brain. According to Anthony Robbins, author of the best-sellers *Unlimited Power* and *Awaken the Giant Within,* "The quality of your life is equal to the quality of the questions you habitually ask yourself." Robbins's opinion is based on the belief that whatever question you ask your brain, you will get an answer. One of the most powerful ways of improving the quality of your life is to improve the quality of your self-talk, particularly the questions you habitually ask yourself.

Let me give you some examples of the questions that my patients with depression ask themselves: "Why am I *always* so depressed?" "Why am I *never* happy?" "Why do things *always* go wrong for me?" "Why do bad things *always* happen to me?" "What is wrong with me?"

First of all, do you notice the permanence in these questions? Terms such as *never* and *always* are seldom true. Yet, I *always* ask my patients questions that challenge their use of *always* and *never*. Usually I will ask them questions such as "Are you *always* depressed?" "Is there *ever* any time that you are not depressed?" "Have you ever experienced even a second of happiness?" "Do things *always* go bad for you?" "Is there anything in your life that has ever gone right?" Their answers to these questions help them realize that terms such as *never* and *always* just do not apply. As to their question What is wrong with me? I tell them that nothing is wrong with them, we simply need to work on tuning up their attitude and physiology. I point out to them that their self-talk and habitual questions are making a powerful imprint on their subconscious and that we need to utilize positive affirmations and questions in order to promote healing. I ask them, "What are some better questions that you can ask of yourself regarding your mood?" I ask them, "If you had happiness and high energy levels right now, what would it feel like?" If they say, "I don't know," then I ask them to imagine what it would feel like. If they can imagine it, then I know they can achieve it. To help them get into the habit of asking empowering questions, I give them the following questions:

The Morning Questions

1. What am I most happy about in my life right now?

   Why does that make me happy?
   How does that make me feel?

2. What am I most excited about in my life right now?

   Why does that make me excited?
   How does that make me feel?

3. What am I most grateful about in my life right now?

   Why does that make me grateful?
   How does that make me feel?

4. What am I enjoying most in my life right now?

   What about that do I enjoy?
   How does that make me feel?

5. What am I committed to in my life right now?

   Why am I committed to that?
   How does that make me feel?

6. Whom do I love? (Starting close and moving out)

Who loves me?

7. What must I do today to achieve my long-term goal?

The Evening Questions

1. What have I given today?

In what ways have I been a giver today?

2. What did I learn today?

3. What did I do today to reach my long-term goal?

4. In what ways was today a perfect day?

5. Repeat the morning questions.

The Problem or Challenge Questions

1. What is right/great about this problem?

2. What is not perfect yet?

3. What am I willing to do to make it the way I want?

4. How can I enjoy doing the things necessary to make it the way I want it?

The habitual asking of these questions is powerful in reprogramming the subconscious mind. It sounds simple and it is, but it really works. Give it a try for one month and I'll guarantee that you'll have a greater enjoyment and passion for life.

Final Comments

One last tip on learning how to become more optimistic is seeking the help of a qualified professional. There are a number of psychological therapies that can be quite useful in helping eliminate depression. The therapy that I feel has the most merit and support in the medical literature is called cognitive therapy. In fact cognitive therapy has been shown to be equally as effective as antidepressant drugs in treating moderate depression.[6] However, while there is a high rate of relapse of depression when drugs are used, the relapse rate for cognitive therapy is much lower. People taking drugs for depression tend to have to stay on them for the rest of their lives. That is not the case with cognitive therapy because the patient is taught new skills to deal with depression.[7]

Psychologists and other mental health specialists trained in cognitive therapy seek to change the way the depressed person consciously thinks about failure, defeat, loss, and helplessness. Cognitive therapists employ five basic tactics.

First they help patients recognize the negative automatic thoughts that flit through consciousness at the times when the patient feels the worst. The second tactic is disputing the negative thoughts by focusing on contrary evidence. The third tactic is teaching the patient a different explanation to dispute the negative automatic thoughts. The fourth tactic involves learning how to avoid rumination (the constant churning of a thought in one's mind) by helping the patient better control his or her thoughts. The final tactic is questioning depression-causing negative thoughts and beliefs and replacing them with empowering positive thoughts and beliefs.

Cognitive therapy does not involve the long, drawn-out process of psychoanalysis. It is a solution-oriented psychotherapy designed at helping the patient learn skills to improve the quality of his or her life. If your thought processes are in need of a little rewiring, please consult a mental health specialist who practices cognitive therapy.

Chapter 3

Ruling Out
an Organic Cause

Depression will often be due to an underlying organic or physiological cause. My goal in this chapter is to take you through the diagnostic process that I follow in my medical practice when I am faced with a patient I think may be depressed. What I want to make sure that I accomplish is to rule out or eliminate easily reversible organic causes of depression. I utilize the same diagnostic approach in virtually every patient who is suffering from a psychological or neurological disturbance. Table 3.1 lists some of the identifiable causes of depression that I will try to rule out.

Table 3.1 Organic and Physiological Causes of Depression

Preexisting Physical Condition
  Diabetes
  Heart disease
  Lung disease
  Rheumatoid arthritis
  Chronic inflammation
  Chronic pain
  Cancer
  Liver disease
  Multiple sclerosis

  Premenstrual syndrome
  Stress/low adrenal function
  Heavy metals
  Food allergies
  Hypothyroidism
  Hypoglycemia
  Nutritional deficiencies
  Sleep disturbances

Drugs
  Prescription
    Antihypertensives
    Anti-inflammatory agents
    Birth control pills
    Antihistamines
    Corticosteroids
    Tranquilizers and
      sedatives

Depression is often a side effect of a person's medical condition or the prescription drugs he or she may be taking. Common drugs associated with depression include corticosteroids, beta-blockers, and other antihypertensive medications. In addition substances not often considered drugs, such as oral contraceptives, alcohol, caffeine, and cigarettes, can cause depression. All these drugs disrupt the normal balance between the monoamine systems in the brain. If you are taking any medication, consult a *Physician's Desk Reference* or your pharmacist about the possibility that the drug is causing depression as a side effect. For most health conditions there are natural medicines that will produce better results than drugs without side effects. Please consult my book *Natural Alternatives to Over-the-Counter and Prescription Drugs* (William Morrow, 1994).

Clinical Evaluation of the Depressed Individual

To make the best use of time in my office, I first utilize a very detailed patient questionnaire to provide me information on the patient's medical history along with a series of questions organized in categories of body function. Answers to these questions provide a detailed review of different body systems. Some of the sections from the questionnaire that I use are contained in this chapter.

Before I see a patient for the first time, I look over the questionnaire to familiarize myself with the case and formulate a series of questions to gain more information if needed. I then sit down with the patient and get to know him on a personal level before asking him about his medical condition. My goal is to identify as many identifiable factors as possible that may be contributing to a less-than-optimal state of health. Sometimes this is really easy, other times it is more difficult.

When the primary complaint is depression, I usually perform laboratory studies to rule out some easily reversible causes of depression. For example, for menstruating women I will typically recommend a sensitive indicator of iron status (the serum ferritin test) along with a complete blood count (CBC) and chemistry panel. For men I'll order just the CBC and chemistry panel. I have the laboratory freeze the serum in case there are any further tests needed based on the results of the CBC and chemistry panel rather than having the patient subjected to another blood draw (I don't like needles either). I try to avoid ordering expensive laboratory tests unless they are absolutely necessary. But, as you will see, there are a number of laboratory tests that are useful in ruling out an organic cause of depression.

Table 3.2 Recommended Initial Blood Tests in Depressed Patients

Complete Blood Count

WBC count	RDW
RBC count	Platelet count
RBC morphology	Differential
Hemoglobin	Neutrophils
MCV	Lymphocytes
MCH	Monocytes
MCHC	Eosinophils

Erythrocyte Sedimentation Rate

Chemistry Panel

Sodium	Anion gap
Potassium	Protein
Chloride	Albumin
CO_2	Globulin

A/G ratio

LDH

AST (SGOT)

ALT (SGPT)

Bilirubin

    Total

    Direct

Alkaline phosphatase

Calcium

Phosphorus

Uric acid

BUN/Creatinine

Glucose

Cholesterol

Triglycerides

Thyroid panel

    T3 uptake

    Thyroxine

    Free thyroxine index

Ferritin (women only)

I may order additional tests based on the results found during the patient interview or from the patient questionnaire. Typically the patient questionnaire or medical history will indicate whether I need to rule out:

Nutritional deficiency

Premenstrual syndrome

Stress and low adrenal function

Heavy metal toxicity

Food allergies

Hypothyroidism

Hypoglycemia

Lifestyle factors

The methods for ruling out all of these conditions except lifestyle factors (discussed in Chapter 4) are provided below.

Nutritional Deficiency

I do not order any tests to rule out nutritional deficiency. Instead I examine a patient's diet diary (a list of all food and drink consumed for at least three days). Tests are not necessary because results will not alter treatment. The guidelines given in Chapter 5 are going to be prescribed regardless.

Premenstrual Syndrome

Premenstrual syndrome (PMS) is a recurrent condition of menstruating women characterized by troublesome symptoms seven to fourteen days before menstruation. Symptoms can include such problems as anxiety, irritability, mood swings, sugar cravings, insomnia, headache, breast tenderness, and water retention. PMS is estimated to affect between 30 and 40 percent of all menstruating women.

Table 3.3 Signs and Symptoms of the Premenstrual Syndrome

Behavioral

    Nervousness, anxiety, and irritability

    Mood swings and mild-to-severe personality change

    Fatigue, lethargy, and depression

Gastrointestinal
    Abdominal bloating
    Diarrhea and/or constipation
    Change in appetite (usually craving of sugar)

Female
    Tender and enlarged breasts
    Uterine cramping
    Altered libido

General
    Headache
    Backache
    Acne
    Swelling of fingers and ankles

Although there is a wide spectrum of symptoms, there are common hormonal patterns in PMS patients when compared with symptom-free control groups: Plasma estrogens are elevated and plasma progesterone levels are reduced five to ten days before menses; prolactin levels are elevated in most, but not all PMS patients; follicle stimulating hormone (FSH) levels are elevated six to nine days prior to the onset of menses; aldosterone levels are marginally elevated two to eight days prior to the onset of menses; and hypothyroidism is common.[1]

These hormonal changes appear to be the result of dietary and nutritional factors. Women with PMS tend to consume a less healthful diet compared with women without

PMS. For example, compared with symptom-free women, PMS patients consume: 275% more refined sugar, 79% more dairy products, 78% more sodium, 53% less iron, 77% less manganese, and 52% less zinc.[2] The high consumption of sugar is particularly incriminating. One study revealed that consumption of foods and beverages that are high in sugar content was the major factor in the likelihood of having PMS.[3] The results of the evaluation of 853 women also revealed that chocolate, alcohol, and fruit juice consumption was highest among women with the most severe PMS symptoms.

The use of vitamin and mineral supplements has been shown to be significantly higher in women without PMS than in women with PMS.[2] In one study twelve of fourteen women without PMS took nutritional supplements. By contrast only six of thirty-nine patients with PMS used nutritional supplements on a regular basis. When compared with normal women, the calculated intake of selected nutrients by the PMS patients was much lower—only 2.2% as much for thiamine, 2.2% for riboflavin, 16.7% for niacin, 8.7% for pantothenic acid, and 2.7% for pyridoxine. PMS patients given a multivitamin and mineral supplement containing high doses of magnesium and pyridoxine have been shown to experience a tremendous reduction in PMS symptoms.[4]

Vitamin B_6 and magnesium are very important in the treatment of PMS. Numerous studies have shown impressive effects when these nutrients are given individually. For example in one double-blind cross-over trial, 84 percent of women with PMS had a lower symptom score during the B_6

treatment period.[5] In a double-blind study with magnesium supplementation, magnesium was shown to dramatically relieve PMS mood changes.[6] However, although these nutrients are effective when given alone, better results are probably achieved when these nutrients are provided in a nutritional supplement program as described in Chapter 5. Other nutrients, such as essential fatty acids, vitamin E, and other B-complex vitamins, have also shown good results in relieving PMS symptoms.

In general, along with a good nutritional supplementation plan, here are the key dietary recommendations for PMS:

- Limit consumption of refined carbohydrates (sugar, honey, white flour, etc.) and other concentrated carbohydrates, such as maple syrup, dried fruit, and fruit juice
- Increase protein intake, particularly from vegetable sources such as legumes
- Decrease milk and dairy products
- Decrease intake of fats, especially natural and synthetically saturated fats
- Supplement the diet with one tablespoon of flaxseed oil daily
- Increase green leafy vegetables, except brassica family foods (cabbage, brussels sprouts, and cauliflower)
- Restrict alcohol and tobacco use
- Restrict intake of caffeine (coffee, tea, chocolate, and caffeine-containing foods and beverages)

Stress and Adrenal Function

Stress is a major factor to consider in the depressed individual. To determine the role that stress may play, I rely a lot on my clinical judgment. I also utilize a popular method of rating stress levels—the Social Readjustment Rating Scale, developed by Holmes and Rahe.[7] The scale was originally designed to predict the likelihood of a person getting a serious disease due to stress. Various life-change events are numerically rated according to their potential for causing disease. Notice that even events commonly viewed as positive, such as an outstanding personal achievement, carry with them stress.

Table 3.4 Social Readjustment Rating Scale

Rank	Life Event	Mean Value
1	Death of spouse	100
2	Divorce	73
3	Marital separation	65
4	Jail term	63
5	Death of a close family member	63
6	Personal injury or illness	53
7	Marriage	50
8	Fired at work	47
9	Marital reconciliation	45

Rank	Life Event	Mean Value
10	Retirement	45
11	Change in health of a family member	44
12	Pregnancy	40
13	Sex difficulties	39
14	Gain of a new family member	39
15	Business adjustment	39
16	Change in financial state	38
17	Death of a close friend	37
18	Change to different line of work	36
19	Change in number of arguments with spouse	35
20	Large mortgage	31
21	Foreclosure of mortgage or loan	30
22	Change in responsibilities at work	29
23	Son or daughter leaving home	29
24	Trouble with in-laws	29
25	Outstanding personal achievement	28
26	Wife begins or stops work	26
27	Begin or end school	26
28	Change in living conditions	25
29	Revision of personal habits	24
30	Trouble with boss	23
31	Change in work hours or conditions	20
32	Change in residence	20
33	Change in schools	20
34	Change in recreation	19
35	Change in church activities	19

Rank	Life Event	Mean Value
36	Change in social activities	18
37	Small mortgage	17
38	Change in sleeping habits	16
39	Change in number of family get-togethers	15
40	Change in eating habits	15
41	Vacation	13
42	Christmas	12
43	Minor violations of the law	11

INTERPRETING YOUR SCORE

The standard interpretation of the Social Readjustment Rating scale is that a total of 200 or more units in one year is considered to be predictive of the likelihood of getting a serious disease. However, rather than using the scale solely to predict the likelihood of the patient getting a serious disease, I utilize the scale as an opportunity to gain insight into a person's stress level. Not everyone reacts to stressful events in the same way. I utilize the scale as a rough indicator of a person's stress level.

In most patients where I suspect that stress is a major factor, I will often perform a study called the adrenal stress index. This test measures the level of the adrenal hormones cortisol and dehydroepiandrosterone (DHEA) in the saliva. Your physician can order these tests through virtually any commercial laboratory. The laboratory that I use for this test is Diagnos-Techs (1–800–878–3787). Typically what is found in depressed individuals is an elevated morning cortisol level and a decreased DHEA level. The effects of increased cortisol levels can be depression, mania, nervousness, insomnia, and schizophrenia. Elevated cortisol levels are a well-recognized feature of depression.[8]

One of the key effects of cortisol on mood is related to activating an enzyme (tryptophan oxygenase). When activated, this enzyme results in less tryptophan being delivered to the brain. Since the level of serotonin in the brain is dependent upon how much tryptophan is delivered to the brain, cortisol dramatically reduces the level of serotonin and melatonin (discussed in Chapter 10).[9] In addition, cortisol also "down regulates" serotonin receptors in the brain, making them less sensitive to the serotonin that is available. Elevated cortisol levels are a major factor to rule out in depressed patients.

Here is what I recommend to restore proper adrenal function:

- Develop a regular exercise program.
- Perform for at least ten minutes twice daily a relaxation technique such as meditation, prayer, biofeedback, and self-hypnosis.
- Consume a diet rich in potassium and low in sodium. This dietary recommendation can be achieved easily by increasing the amounts of whole grains, legumes, vegetables, and fruits while reducing the amount of salt and prepared foods.
- Take a high-potency multiple vitamin and mineral formula according to the guidelines given in Chapter 5.
- Take a high-quality *Panax ginseng* extract.

In regard to the last recommendation, *Panax ginseng* (Chinese or Korean ginseng) has been shown to exert many beneficial effects on the adrenal glands and stress response, including an ability to lower elevated cortisol levels.[10] However, in order to gain the benefits of ginseng, it is important to select a high-quality product. The best preparations are extracts that have been standardized for ginsenoside content and ratio to ensure optimum pharmacological effect. The extracts not only are standardized for total ginsenoside content but also for the ratio of ginsenoside $R_{g1}:R_{b1}$ (1:2 is considered ideal). The typical dose (taken one to three times daily) for general tonic effects should contain a ginsenoside content of at least 5 mg. For example, the dosage for a standardized *Panax ginseng* extract containing a 5% ginsenoside content would be 100 mg one to three times daily. As each individual's response to ginseng is unique, it is best to begin at lower doses and increase gradually. Too much ginseng may cause a number of side effects, including anxiety, irritability, nervousness, insomnia, hypertension, breast pain, and menstrual changes. If any of these side effects appear, the dosage should be reduced or the product should be discontinued.

Heavy-Metal Toxicity

Toxic substances are everywhere in our environment. Heavy metals (lead, mercury, cadmium, arsenic, nickel, and aluminum) as well as solvents (cleaning materials, formaldehyde, toluene, benzene, etc.), pesticides, and herbicides have an affinity to nervous tissue. The outcome is that these toxic substances can become concentrated in the brain. As a result a variety of psychological and neurological symptoms can occur including depression, headaches, mental confusion, mental illness, tingling in extremities, abnormal nerve reflexes, and other signs of impaired nervous system function.[11]

A hair mineral analysis is a good screening test for heavy-metal toxicity. If the hair mineral analysis is inconclusive, a more sensitive indicator is the eight-hour lead mobilization test. This test employs the chelating agent EDTA (edetate calcium disodium) and measures the level of lead excreted in the urine for a period of eight hours after the injection of EDTA. The lead mobilization test must be performed by a licensed physician.

In the United States the typical person has more lead and other heavy metals in his or her body than is compatible with health. It is conservatively estimated that up to 25 percent of the United States population suffers from heavy-metal poisoning to some extent. The lead comes primarily from industrial sources such as well-leaded gasoline. Each year in the United States more than 600,000 tons of lead is being dumped into the atmosphere, from which it is inhaled or ingested. Other common sources of heavy metals include: lead from the solder in tin cans, pesticide sprays, and cooking utensils; cadmium and lead from cigarette smoke; mercury from dental fillings, contaminated fish, and cosmetics; and aluminum from antacids and cookware. Some professions with extremely high exposure include: battery makers, gasoline station attendants, printers, roofers, dentists, and jewelers.

Here are my recommendations to help eliminate heavy metals from the body:

- Increase the consumption of foods rich in water-soluble fibers such as pears, apples, legumes, and oat bran.
- Eat one serving of cruciferous vegetables (broccoli, cabbage, brussels sprouts) three times daily.
- Consume foods rich in sulfur such as onions, garlic, and legumes.
- Eliminate alcohol, sugar, saturated fats, drugs, and other substances that impair detoxification.
- Take a high-potency multiple vitamin and mineral formula as described in Chapter 5.
- Take a nutritional formula that supplies choline, methionine, and inositol, such as Liv-A-Tox (Enzymatic Therapy) or Lipotropic Complex (Nature's Life), according to label instructions.
- Take 1,000 mg of vitamin C three times daily.
- Take 1–2 tablespoons of a fiber supplement at night before retiring. The best fiber sources are the water-soluble fibers such as powdered psyllium seed husks, guar gum, oat bran, and so forth.

Food Allergies

Depression and fatigue have been linked to food allergies for over sixty-five years. In 1930 the famous allergist Dr. Albert Rowe used the term *allergic toxemia* to describe a syndrome that included the symptoms of depression, fatigue, muscle and joint aches, drowsiness, difficulty in concentration, and nervousness.[12] Although that term is not used anymore, food allergies still play a major role in many people with depression. Food allergies are the leading cause of most undiagnosed symptoms, and it is estimated that as high as at least 60 percent of the American population suffers from symptoms associated with food reactions.[13]

Table 3.5 Symptoms and Diseases Commonly Associated with Food Allergy

System	Symptoms and Diseases
Mental/emotional	Anxiety, depression, hyperactivity, inability to concentrate, insomnia, irritability, mental confusion, personality change, seizures
Gastrointestinal	Canker sores, celiac disease, chronic diarrhea, duodenal ulcer, gas, gastritis, irritable colon, malabsorption, ulcerative colitis
Genitourinary	Bed-wetting, chronic bladder infections, nephrosis
Immune	Chronic infections, frequent ear infections
Musculoskeletal	Bursitis, joint pain, low back pain
Respiratory	Asthma, chronic bronchitis, wheezing
Skin	Acne, eczema, hives, itching, skin rash
Miscellaneous	Arrhythmia, edema, fainting, fatigue, headache, hypoglycemia, itchy nose or throat, migraines, sinusitis

Food allergies, as well as respiratory tract allergies, are also characterized by the following signs:

Dark circles under the eyes (allergic shiners)
Puffiness under the eyes
Horizontal creases in the lower lid
Chronic fluid retention
Chronic swollen glands

There are two basic categories of tests commonly used to diagnose food allergies: (a) food challenge; and (b) laboratory methods. Each has its advantages. Food-challenge methods require no additional expense, but they do require a great deal of motivation. Laboratory procedures, such as blood tests, can provide immediate identification of suspected allergens, but are more expensive.

The standard food-challenge method involves the use of the elimination (also known as oligoantigenic) diet followed by food reintroduction. In the elimination-diet method the person is placed on a limited diet; commonly eaten foods are eliminated and replaced with low-allergenic foods. The standard elimination diet consists of lamb, chicken, potatoes, rice, banana, apple, and a cabbage-family vegetable (cabbage, brussels sprouts, broccoli, etc.). The individual stays on this limited diet for at least one week and up to one month. If the symptoms are related to food sensitivity, they will typically disappear by the fifth or sixth day of the diet. If the symptoms do not disappear, it is possible that a reaction to a food in the elimination diet is responsible, in which case an even more restricted diet must be utilized.

After symptoms have disappeared, individual foods are reintroduced at a rate of one new food every two days. If a person is allergic to the reintroduced food, it typically produces a more severe or recognizable symptom. A careful, detailed record must be maintained describing when foods were reintroduced and what symptoms appeared upon reintroduction.

For many people, elimination diets offer the most viable means of detection. Because one can sometimes dramatically experience the effects of food reactions, motivation to eliminate the food can be high. The downside of this procedure is that it is time-consuming and requires discipline and motivation. Laboratory tests can now provide immediate feedback.

Food allergies can now be easily identified by the use of special blood tests that measure both IgE and IgG type food allergies. Skin scratch tests are not suitable for detecting food allergies because they only test for IgE type allergies, which account for only 10 to 15 percent of all food allergies.[13] The blood tests are extremely convenient and relatively accurate. The downside is that they also tend to be expensive. In my practice I utilize the food allergy panel from Meridian Valley Clinical Laboratory (1-206-859-8700). It measures both IgE and IgG antibodies, tests for over one hundred different foods, comes with detailed dietary instructions, and is reasonably priced at about $120.

Hypothyroidism

The first symptom observed in hypothyroidism (low thyroid function) is depression, as the brain appears to be extremely sensitive to low thyroid levels.[14] Hypothyroidism is often overlooked by many physicians because they rely on blood measurements of thyroid hormone levels as the method of diagnosis. While blood measurements are suitable in diagnosing severe deficiency of thyroid hormones, for diagnosing milder forms of hypothyroidism, functional tests such the basal body temperature (the temperature of the body at rest) and Achilles reflex time (reflexes are slowed in hypothyroidism) are more sensitive. As mild hypothyroidism is the most common form of hypothyroidism, the majority of people with hypothyroidism are going undiagnosed.[15]

Undiagnosed hypothyroidism is a serious concern, as failure to treat an underlying condition such as hypothyroidism will reduce the effectiveness of every other measure designed to increase energy levels. It is kind of like trying to run your car without a fuel pump. There may be plenty of gas in the tank, but it is simply not being delivered to the engine.

In my clinical practice, when I suspect hypothyroidism, I'll have the patient take his or her basal body temperature—the temperature of the body at rest. The basal body temperature is the most sensitive functional test of thyroid function.[15] A simple method for taking your basal body temperature is detailed below.

TAKING YOUR BASAL BODY TEMPERATURE

Your basal body temperature reflects your resting metabolic rate, which is largely determined by hormones secreted by the thyroid gland. The function of the thyroid gland can be determined by simply measuring your basal body temperature. All that is needed is a thermometer.

Procedure

1. Shake down the thermometer to below 95°F and place it by your bed before going to sleep at night.
2. On waking, place the thermometer in your armpit for a full ten minutes. It is important to make as little movement as possible. Lying and resting with your eyes closed is best. Do not get up until the ten-minute test is completed.
3. After ten minutes, read and record the temperature and date.
4. Record the temperature for at least three mornings (preferably at the same time of day). Menstruating women must perform the test on the second, third, and fourth days of menstruation. Men and postmenopausal women can perform the test at any time.

Interpretation

Your basal body temperature should be between 97.6° and 98.2°. Low basal body temperatures are quite common and may reflect hypothyroidism. In addition to fatigue, common signs and symptoms of hypothyroidism are low basal body temperature, depression, difficulty in losing weight, dry skin, headaches, menstrual problems, recurrent infections, constipation, and sensitivity to cold.

High basal body temperatures (above 98.6°) are less common, but may be evidence of hyperthyroidism. Common signs and symptoms of hyperthyroidism include bulging eyeballs, fast pulse, hyperactivity, inability to gain weight, insomnia, irritability, menstrual problems, and nervousness.

TREATING HYPOTHYROIDISM

In all but its mildest forms, the medical treatment of hypothyroidism requires the use of prescription desiccated thyroid or synthetic thyroid hormone. Although synthetic hormones have become popular, many physicians (particularly naturopathic physicians) still prefer the use of desiccated natural thyroid, complete with all thyroid hormones. At this time it appears that thyroid hormone replacement is necessary in the majority of people with hypothyroidism.

The thyroid extracts sold in health food stores are required by the Food and Drug Administration (FDA) to be thyroxine-free. However, it is nearly impossible to remove all the hormone from the gland. In other words, think of health food store thyroid preparations as milder forms of desiccated natural thyroid. If you have very mild hypothyroidism, these preparations may provide enough support to help you with your thyroid problem. Follow the manufacturer's recommendations as provided on the product's label. Use your basal body temperature to determine effectiveness of the product.

Hypoglycemia

Hypoglycemia (low blood sugar) is another common cause of depression.[16] Hypoglycemia is a result of faulty carbohydrate (sugar) metabolism. The body strives to maintain blood sugar (glucose) levels within a narrow range primarily to assure the brain a constant and even supply of glucose, the brain's primary source of energy. Typically symptoms of hypoglycemia affect the brain first.

When glucose levels are low, as occurs during hypoglycemia, the brain does not function properly. Symptoms of hypoglycemia can range from mild to severe and include such things as depression, anxiety, irritability, and other psychological disturbances; fatigue; headache; blurred vision; excessive sweating; mental confusion; incoherent speech; bizarre behavior; and convulsions.

The association between hypoglycemia and depression is largely ignored by most physicians—they simply never even consider it as a possibility despite the fact that several studies have shown hypoglycemia to be very common in depressed individuals.[15] There is no explanation for this oversight by so many physicians, especially since dietary therapy (usually simply eliminating refined carbohydrate from the diet) is occasionally all that is needed for effective therapy in patients that have depression due to reactive hypoglycemia.

The standard method of diagnosing hypoglycemia is the oral glucose tolerance test (GTT). It is used in the diagnosis of both hypoglycemia and diabetes, although it is rarely required for the latter. After the subject has fasted for at least twelve hours, a baseline blood glucose measurement is made. Then the subject is given a very sweet liquid containing glucose to drink. Blood sugar levels are rechecked at thirty minutes, one hour, and then hourly for up to six hours. Basically, if blood sugar levels rise to a level greater than 200 mg/dl, it indicates diabetes. If levels fall below 50 mg/dl, it indicates reactive hypoglycemia. Hypoglycemia can also be diagnosed if there is a decrease of 20 mg or more from the fasting level after four hours. A diagnosis of probable reactive hypoglycemia is made if there is a decrease of 10 to 20 mg from the fasting level after four hours.

Because many of the symptoms linked to hypoglycemia can be a result of increases in insulin, it has been recommended that insulin be measured at the same time, since symptoms often correlate better with elevations in insulin than with glucose levels. This test is called the glucose-insulin tolerance test (G-ITT) and is a much more sensitive indicator of hypoglycemia than the standard GTT.[17]

Despite the GTT and G-ITT being the standard diagnostic tools for hypoglycemia, I rarely order them. The reason is that I have found the most useful measure of diagnosing hypoglycemia is a patient questionnaire that assesses symptoms often attributable to hypoglycemia.

Hypoglycemia Questionnaire

	No = 0	Mild = 1	Moderate = 2	Severe = 3
Crave sweets	0	1	2	3
Irritable if a meal is missed	0	1	2	3
Feel tired or weak if a meal is missed	0	1	2	3
Dizziness when standing suddenly	0	1	2	3
Frequent headaches	0	1	2	3
Poor memory (forgetful) or concentration	0	1	2	3
Feel tired an hour or so after eating	0	1	2	3
Heart palpitations	0	1	2	3
Feel shaky at times	0	1	2	3
Afternoon fatigue	0	1	2	3
Vision blurs on occasion	0	1	2	3
Depression or mood swings	0	1	2	3

	No = 0	Mild = 1	Moderate = 2	Severe = 3
Overweight	0	1	2	3
Frequently anxious or nervous	0	1	2	3
Total				_____

Scoring:

> Less than 5 = hypoglycemia is not likely a factor
> 6–15 = hypoglycemia is a likely factor
> Greater than 15 = hypoglycemia is extremely likely

Eliminating the intake of refined sugar and limiting the intake of fruit is often all that is needed to reestablish proper control of blood sugar levels. In addition, taking supplemental chromium (200–400 mcg per day), as either chromium polynicotinate or chromium picolinate, can be very useful, as chromium is critical to proper blood sugar control.

Final Comments

As detailed above, there are a number of organic causes of depression that must be ruled out. In many cases there will likely be more than one identifiable cause. If so, each factor must be effectively dealt with. A good physician can go a long way in helping identify some of these easily overlooked factors. Please take this book along with you when visiting your physician if you would like him or her to rule out these factors that often contribute to depression. Successful treatment of depression with natural measures requires identification and control of underlying factors.

Chapter 4

Lifestyle Factors
in Depression

M ost of the health problems of Americans are related to lifestyle and dietary practices. Of particular detriment to health are the addiction to nicotine, caffeine, and other stimulants. According to Joseph Beasley, M.D., the primary investigator involved in the famous *Kellogg Report: The Impact of Nutrition, Environment, and Lifestyle on Illness in America,* the United States is a nation of addicts. The spectrum of addiction ranges on one end from the typical American who "can't get started in the morning" without a cup of coffee to the other end with the strung-out crack addict. Dr. Beasley offers some considerable evidence to support his belief:[1]

- Americans consume 450 million cups of coffee each day.
- Half of the population between the ages of thirty and sixty define themselves as coffee drinkers.
- At least 15 million Americans drink six or more cups of coffee each day.
- Of American adults, 30 percent smoke at least half a pack of cigarettes each day.
- At least 10 percent of the population is addicted to alcohol.
- Anywhere from 24 to 33 percent of the population consume four to thirteen drinks daily.
- One third of high school seniors report "binge drinking" (five or more drinks in a row) at least once in the last two weeks.
- Every year Americans swallow more than 5 billion tranquilizers, such as Valium and Xanax.
- Cocaine addiction afflicts at least 2.2 million persons, with about 1 percent of the United States population using cocaine at least once per week.

In many instances people claim that they smoke, drink alcohol, or take drugs because it calms them. In reality these substances actually complicate matters. The relaxation and/or chemical high from these drugs is short-lived and ultimately leads to adding even more stress to the system. Individuals suffering from depression or other psychological conditions must absolutely stop smoking, drinking alcohol, and ingesting coffee and other sources of caffeine.

Smoking and Depression

Cigarette smoking is one of the major factors contributing to premature death in the United States. Health experts have determined that cigarette smoking is the single major cause of cancer death in the United States. Cigarette smokers have total, overall cancer death rates twice that of nonsmokers. The greater the number of cigarettes smoked, the greater the risk.[2]

Smoking also increases the risk of death from heart attack and stroke. In fact, according to the U.S. Surgeon General, "Cigarette smoking should be considered the most important risk factor for coronary heart disease." Statistical evidence reveals a three- to fivefold increase in the risk of coronary artery disease in smokers compared with nonsmokers. The more cigarettes smoked and the longer the period of years a person has smoked, the greater the risk of dying from a heart attack or stroke. Overall the average smoker dies seven to eight years sooner than the nonsmoker.[2]

Cigarette smoking is also a significant factor in depression. Central to the effect of nicotine is the stimulation of adrenal hormone, including cortisol, secretion. The role of cortisol in depression was discussed on page 67. Elevated cortisol levels significantly inhibit serotonin activity in the brain and lead to depression.

Cigarette smoking also leads to a relative vitamin C deficiency, as the vitamin C is utilized to detoxify the cigarette smoke. Low levels of vitamin C in the brain can result in depression and hysteria.[3]

If you smoke, you absolutely must stop. Here are ten tips to help you stop:

1. List all the reasons why you want to quit smoking, and review them daily.
2. Set a specific day to quit, tell at least ten friends that you are going to quit smoking, and then DO IT!
3. Throw away all cigarettes, butts, matches, and ashtrays.
4. Use substitutes. Instead of smoking, chew on raw vegetables, fruits, or gum. If your fingers seem empty, play with a pencil.
5. Realize that forty million Americans have quit. If they can do it, so can you!
6. Visualize yourself as a nonsmoker with a fatter pocketbook, pleasant breath, unstained teeth, and the satisfaction that comes from being in control of your life.
7. Join a support group. Call the local American Cancer Society and ask for referrals. You are not alone.
8. When you need to relax, perform deep-breathing exercises rather than reaching for a cigarette.
9. Avoid situations that you associate with smoking.
10. Take each hour and every day one at a time. Each day reward yourself in a positive way. Buy yourself something with the money you've saved or plan a special reward as a celebration for quitting.

Alcohol and Depression

Individuals with depression must avoid alcohol. Alcohol is a brain depressant. It also increases adrenal hormone output, interferes with many brain cell processes, and disrupts normal sleep cycles. Alcohol ingestion also leads to hypoglycemia. The resultant drop in blood sugar produces a craving for sugar because it can quickly elevate blood sugar. Unfortunately increased sugar consumption ultimately aggravates the hypoglycemia. Hypoglycemia aggravates the mental and emotional problems of the alcoholic.

If you think you may have a drinking problem, seek help. Contact your local Alcoholics Anonymous or similar social program.

Caffeine and Depression

Caffeine must also be avoided by patients with depression. Caffeine is a stimulant. A person's response to caffeine will vary; however, people prone to feeling depressed or anxious tend to be especially sensitive to caffeine. The term *caffeinism* is used to describe a clinical syndrome similar to generalized anxiety and panic disorders that includes such symptoms as depression, nervousness, palpitations, irritability, and recurrent headache.[4]

Several studies have looked at caffeine intake and depression. For example, one study found that among healthy college students moderate and high coffee drinkers scored higher on a depression scale than did low users. Interestingly the moderate and high coffee drinkers also tended to have significantly lower academic performance.[5] Several other studies have shown that depressed patients tend to consume fairly high amounts of caffeine (e.g., greater than 700 mg per day).[6] The intake of caffeine has been positively correlated with the degree of mental illness in psychiatric patients. In other words the more caffeine that is consumed, the greater the mental illness in these patients.[7]

The combination of caffeine and refined sugar seem to be even worse than either substance consumed alone. Several studies have found an association between this combination and depression. In one of the most interesting studies twenty-one women and two men responded to an advertisement requesting volunteers "who feel depressed and don't know why, often feel tired even though they sleep a lot, are very moody, and generally seem to feel bad most of the time." After baseline psychological testing, the subjects were placed on a caffeine- and sucrose-free diet for one week. Subjects who reported substantial improvement were retested and were challenged in a double-blind fashion. The subjects either took a capsule containing caffeine and a Kool-Aid drink sweetened with sugar or they took a capsule containing cellulose and a Kool-Aid drink sweetened with Nutrasweet. Each challenge lasted up to six days. About 50 percent of test subjects became depressed during the test period with caffeine and sucrose.[8]

Another study using a format similar to the Kool-Aid study described above found that seven of sixteen depressed patients were found to be depressed with the caffeine and sucrose challenge, but became symptom-free during the caffeine- and sucrose-free diet and cellulose and Nutrasweet test period.[9]

The average American consumes 150–225 mg of caffeine daily, or roughly the amount of caffeine in one to two cups of coffee. Although most people can handle this amount, some people are more sensitive to the effects of caffeine than others. Even small amounts of caffeine, as found in decaffeinated coffee, are enough to affect some people adversely and produce caffeinism. People with depression or any psychological disorder should avoid caffeine completely.

Table 4.1 Caffeine Content of Coffee, Tea, and Selected Soft Drinks

Beverage	Caffeine (mg)
Coffee (7.5 oz cup)	
Drip	115–150
Brewed	80–135
Instant	65–40
Decaffeinated	3–4
Tea (5 oz cup)	
1-min. brew	20
3-min. brew	35
Iced (12 oz)	70

Beverage	Caffeine (mg)
Soft drinks	
Jolt	100
Mountain Dew	54
Tab	47
Coca-Cola	45
Diet Coke	45
Dr Pepper	40
Pepsi-Cola	38
Diet Pepsi	36
7UP	0

If you have been a heavy coffee drinker, be aware that when you quit, you may experience withdrawal symptoms including fatigue, headache, and an intense desire for coffee. Fortunately, this withdrawal period doesn't last more than a day or two.

Exercise and Depression

Regular exercise may be the most powerful natural antidepressant available. In fact, many of the beneficial effects of exercise noted in the prevention of heart disease may be related just as much to its ability to improve mood as improve cardiovascular function.[10] Various community and clinical studies have clearly indicated that exercise has profound antidepressive effects.[11] These studies have shown that increased participation in exercise, sports, and physical activities is strongly associated with decreased symptoms of anxiety (restlessness, tension, etc.), depression (feelings that life is not worthwhile, low spirits, etc.), and malaise (run-down feeling, insomnia, etc.). Furthermore, people who participate in regular exercise have higher self-esteem, feel better, and are much happier compared with people who do not exercise.

Much of the mood-elevating effect of exercise may be attributed to the fact that regular exercise has been shown to increase the level of powerful mood-elevating substances in the brain known as endorphins.[12] These compounds exert effects similar to morphine. In fact, their name (*endo* = endogenous, *-rphins* = morphines) was given to them because of their morphinelike effects. Have you ever heard of the "runner's high?" Well, the reason for the elation that some runners feel when exercising is the rush of endorphins that the exercise promotes.

When endorphin levels are low, depression occurs. Conversely, when endorphin levels are elevated, so is one's mood. In one of the most interesting studies that examined the role of exercise and endorphins in depression, Dennis Lobstein, Ph.D., a professor of exercise psychobiology at the University of New Mexico, compared the beta-endorphin levels and depression profiles of ten joggers versus ten sedentary men of the same age. The ten sedentary men tested out more depressed, perceived greater stress in their lives, had more stress-circulating hormones and lower levels of beta-endorphins. As Dr. Lobstein stated, this "reaffirms that depression is very sensitive to exercise and helps firm up a biochemical link between physical activity and depression."[13]

There have been at least one hundred clinical studies where an exercise program has been used in the treatment of depression. In an analysis of the sixty-four studies prior to 1980, physical fitness training was shown to relieve depression and improve self-esteem and work behavior.[14] Unfortunately, the quality of many of the studies was less than ideal. However, because of the good results noted in the analysis of these studies, there was a flurry of well-designed studies conducted in the 1980s to better determine how effective exercise could be as a therapy. These studies utilized stricter scientific criteria than the earlier ones, yet they produced similar results. It was concluded that exercise can be as effective as other antidepressants, including drugs and psychotherapy.[15] More recently, even stricter studies have further demonstrated that regular exercise is a powerful antidepressant.[16]

The intensity of exercise necessary to gain psychological benefits is less than that required to gain improvement in cardiovascular function, but it still should be performed in the proper training zone. The training zone is determined by your heart rate (pulse). The upper end of the training zone is calculated by subtracting your age from 185. For example, if you are forty years old, your maximum heart rate would be 145. To determine the bottom of the training zone, simply subtract 30 from this number. In the case of a forty-year-old, this would be 115. So the training zone would be a heartbeat between 115 and 145 beats per minute. A minimum of fifteen to twenty minutes of exercising at your training heart rate at least three times a week is necessary to gain any significant psychological as well as cardiovascular benefits. Exercising at the lower end of your training zone for longer periods of time is much better than exercising at a higher intensity for a shorter period of time.

The best exercises are either strength training (weight lifting) or aerobic activities such as walking briskly, jogging, bicycling, cross-country skiing, swimming, aerobic dance, and racquet sports. The important thing is to train with an intensity that will keep your heart rate in the training zone.

Table 4.2 The Benefits of Regular Exercise

Psychological

Provides a natural release for pent-up feelings

Helps reduce tension and anxiety

Improves mental outlook and self-esteem

Helps relieve moderate depression

Improves the ability to handle stress

Stimulates improved mental function

Relaxes and improves sleep

Increases self-esteem

Musculoskeletal System

Increases muscle strength

Increases flexibility of muscles and range of joint motion

Produces stronger bones, ligaments, and tendons

Lessens chance of injury

Enhances posture, poise, and physique

Heart and Blood Vessels
  Lowers resting heart rate
  Strengthens heart function
  Lowers blood pressure
  Improves oxygen delivery throughout the body
  Increases blood supply to muscles
  Enlarges the arteries to the heart

Bodily Processes
  Reduces heart disease risk
  Helps lower blood cholesterol and triglycerides
  Raises HDL, the "good" cholesterol
  Helps improve calcium deposition in bones
  Prevents osteoporosis
  Improves immune function
  Aids digestion and elimination
  Increases lean body mass
  Improves the body's ability to burn dietary fat
  Increases endurance and energy levels
  Increases strength
  Improves blood sugar control
  Reduces risk of diabetes
  Promotes longevity

If you are not currently on a regular exercise program, get medical clearance if you have health problems or if you are over forty years of age. The main concern is the functioning of your heart. Exercise can be quite harmful (even fatal) if your heart is not able to meet the increased demands placed upon it.

It is especially important to see a physician if any of the following applies to you:

Heart disease

Smoking

High blood pressure

Extreme breathlessness with physical exertion

Pain or pressure in chest, arm, teeth, jaw, or neck with exercise

Dizziness or fainting

Abnormal heart action (palpitations or irregular beat)

Regular physical exercise is clearly important to good health, yet less than 20 percent of Americans exercise on a regular basis. Why? Excuses such as lack of time, energy, or motivation are frequently given. Are these excuses valid? How important is your health? How important is regular exercise to your overall health? You must make regular exercise a top priority in your life.

Stress Management

Stress is a term we are all too familiar with. We often think of stress as an outside force, yet it is an internal response to a specific stimulation, known as a *stressor*. A stressor is anything that disturbs body function. It may be psychological, such as job and financial pressure and strong emotions, or physiological, such as exposure to heat or cold, environmental toxins,

toxins produced by microorganisms, or physical trauma.

Psychological stress can produce what is known as the alarm reaction, or fight-or-flight response. The fight-or-flight response is an internal protective measure designed to counteract danger by mobilizing the body's resources for immediate physical activity, either to fight or to run away. The adrenal glands play a key role in the stress response because they secrete adrenaline and other stress-related hormones. These hormones are responsible for many of the feelings of stress as well as the fight-or-flight response. A surge of adrenaline is great if you need to escape from a tiger or some other life-threatening situation. However, if stress is extreme, unusual, or long-lasting, these stress mechanisms can be quite harmful. Stress can also be a problem if a person does not regularly employ a method of stress reduction.

Table 4.3 Conditions Strongly Linked to Psychological Stress

Angina	Hypertension
Asthma	Immune suppression
Autoimmune disease	Irritable bowel syndrome
Cancer	Menstrual irregularities
Cardiovascular disease	Premenstrual tension syndrome
Common cold	drome
Depression	Rheumatoid arthritis
Diabetes (adult-onset—type II)	Ulcerative colitis
Headache	Ulcers

Physical exercise is a great stress reducer and is a necessary component in a comprehensive stress management program. However, passive methods of stress reduction are also extremely important to practice. Relaxation techniques such as meditation, prayer, self-hypnosis, biofeedback, and visualizations should be performed for at least ten to fifteen minutes each day.

Relaxation techniques seek to counteract the results of stress by inducing its opposite—relaxation. Although an individual may relax by simply sleeping, watching television, or reading a book, relaxation techniques are designed specifically to produce the *relaxation response*—a term used to describe the physiological state that Harvard professor and cardiologist Herbert Benson, M.D., describes in his best-selling book, *The Relaxation Response* (William Morrow, 1975).

The physiological effects of the relaxation response are opposite to those seen with stress. In the stress response, the sympathetic nervous system dominates. In the relaxation response, the parasympathetic nervous system dominates. The parasympathetic nervous system controls bodily functions such as digestion, breathing, and heart rate during periods of rest, relaxation, visualization, meditation, and sleep. While the sympathetic nervous system is designed to protect us against immediate danger, the parasympathetic system is designed for repair, maintenance, and restoration of the body.

Producing deep relaxation with any relaxation technique requires learning how to breathe. Have you ever noticed how a baby breathes? With each breath, the baby's abdomen rises and falls because the baby is breathing with its diaphragm, a dome-shaped muscle that separates the chest cavity from the abdominal cavity. If you are like most adults, you tend to fill only your upper chest because you do not utilize the diaphragm. Shallow breathing tends to produce tension and fatigue.

One of the most powerful methods of eliminating stress and producing more energy in the body is breathing with the diaphragm. By using the diaphragm to breathe, a person dramatically changes his or her physiology. Diaphragmatic breathing literally activates the relaxation centers in the brain. Here is a popular technique I use to train people to breathe using their diaphragm:

1. Find a comfortable and quiet place to lie down or sit.
2. Place your feet slightly apart. Place one hand on your abdomen near your navel. Place the other hand on your chest.
3. You will be inhaling through your nose and exhaling through your mouth.
4. Concentrate on your breathing. Note which hand is rising and falling with each breath.
5. Gently exhale most of the air in your lungs.
6. Inhale while slowly counting to 4. As you inhale, slightly extend your abdomen, causing it to rise about one inch. Make sure that you are not moving your chest or shoulders.
7. As you breathe in, imagine the warmed air flowing in. Imagine its warmth flowing to all parts of your body.
8. Pause for one second, then slowly exhale to a count of

4. As you exhale, your abdomen should move inward.

9. As the air flows out, imagine all the tension and stress leaving your body.

10. Repeat the process until a sense of deep relaxation is achieved.

Now that you know how to breathe, the important thing is to remember to breathe with your diaphragm as much as possible—especially during times of increased stress—and to perform a relaxation technique for ten to fifteen minutes each day.

To help get you started, here is an excellent visualization script adapted from *Rituals of Healing: Using Imagery for Health and Wellness* by Jeanne Achterberg, Barbara Dossey, and Leslie Kolkmeier. Use it to promote the relaxation response, overall healing, and general well-being.

Before you begin your imagery journey, find a quiet, comfortable place and give yourself permission to spend fifteen or twenty minutes taking care of yourself. Lie down, or sit with your back and neck completely supported. Allow your chair, or bed, or wherever you are to hold you. Let tension melt away as you bring your attention to your breath, listening to and feeling the in breath, the out breath. . . . [Pause for one minute.] Take a mental journey now, through your body, beginning at the bottom of your feet. Move your attention slowly to the top of your head, letting go of any tightness or restriction you find. [Pause for one or two minutes, or guide yourself through your muscle groups.]

Your mind has just moved through your body, connecting with it, giving it attention, soothing the tense, tired places. Now let your mind move to a still point. Some people find this still point deep within, a place of pure peace and calm. A place of quiet knowing. Let the words *still point* fill your mind, chasing out other thoughts and concerns. Breathe yourself into this quiet place. Quietly, gently find the stillness. [Pause one minute.]

Sit comfortably, with your back straight but relaxed. Focus on your breath and inhale and exhale three times. Then, slowly, begin to inhale.

As you feel the air moving in through your nose and down the back of your throat into your lungs, hear yourself saying, way in the back of your mind, "One." . . . Feel the air moving back out. . . . As the next breath begins to fill your lungs, hear yourself saying, deep inside yourself . . . "Two." . . . Feel the air moving back out. . . . With the next breath in, hear yourself saying, deep inside yourself, "Three." . . . Feel the air moving back out. . . . With the next breath in, hear yourself saying, deep inside yourself, "Four." . . . Feel the air moving back out. . . . Repeat this cycle as many times as you wish. . . . Counting 1 to 4 with your breaths.

With each breath in . . . feel your diaphragm moving down toward your feet . . . and your lower ab-

domen beginning to expand. . . . With each breath out
. . . as your abdomen relaxes . . . feel the muscles in
your neck and shoulders drifting down with gravity . . .
and relaxing even more deeply.

Imagine your body is made of a beautiful, clear
crystalline material. . . . Each time you breathe in, imagine your breath is a healing, colored mist . . . any color
that comes to mind. . . . Feel the healing mist entering
your body through the top of your head and drifting
slowly down inside your crystal-clear body. . . . See and
feel that mist beginning to fill you with relaxation and
calm. . . . Each time you breathe in, imagine that colored mist adding relaxation. . . . Each breath slowly fills
your crystal body with peace and healing. . . . Continue
to see yourself filling with color until your body is completely full of relaxation. . . .

With the next breath in, say to yourself, "I am
breathing . . ." With the breath out, say to yourself,
". . . warmth into my feet." With the next breath in,
say to yourself, "I am breathing . . ." With the breath
out, say to yourself, ". . . warmth into my legs." Continue in this manner, breathing warmth into all parts of
your body. . . . Gradually come back to full awareness
of the room and notice your calmness and relaxation.

This technique can promote a phenomenal sense of deep
relaxation. The stresses of modern living will simply melt
away. Can a regularly performed stress-reduction technique
relieve depression and promote happiness? Yes, according to

reat deal about life in a relatively short period of time.
the things she helped me realize is just how much
ly know how to laugh and play. If you do not have
our own, spend time with your nieces, nephews, or
hood children with whose families you are friendly.
a Big Brother or Big Sister. Investigate local Little
Help out at your church's Sunday school and chil-
ents. Kids can teach us a lot about how to laugh hard
y life.

one study that investigated the impact that a visualization exercise has on happiness.[17] Subjects were enrolled in a Personal
Happiness Enhancement Program (PHEP) and divided into
two groups, both of which received instruction on the PHEP.
Subjects in one experimental group were taught a visualization exercise in addition to the PHEP. A third group, the
control group, received no instruction. At the beginning and
end of the program subjects were tested on various psychological scales for happiness (Happiness Measure, Psychap Inventory, Beck Depression Inventory, and State-Trait Anxiety
Scale). The results of the study found that the meditation-
plus-PHEP group significantly improved on all dependent
measures over both the PHEP-only group and the control
group.

If you find yourself having trouble learning how to relax
or perform visualization exercises, I urge you to consult with
an expert. For an expert in your area, please contact:

The Academy for Guided Imagery
P.O. Box 2070
Mill Valley, CA 94942
1-800-726-2070

Final Comments

A health-promoting lifestyle can go a long way in the treatment of depression. Particularly important is the cessation of
smoking, excessive alcohol consumption, and the intake of

caffeine. These lifestyle changes coupled with regular exercise and the performance of a stress-reduction technique would more than likely produce far better clinical results than Prozac at absolutely no cost.

Another important lifestyle factor that must be mentioned is the injection of humor into life. Laughter may prove to be the most powerful medicine. The benefits of humor have been accepted throughout human history. Humor is widely accepted for its positive physiological and psychological effects in a variety of situations. Humor has also been shown to be an effective tool in psychiatric illness and psychotherapy, especially in severely depressed and suicidal individuals.[18] Recent medical research has also confirmed that laughter[19]

- Plays an active part in the body's release of endorphins and other natural mood-elevating and painkilling chemicals
- Enhances blood flow to the body's extremities and improves cardiovascular function
- Improves the transfer of oxygen and nutrients to internal organs
- Enhances immune function[18]

By laughing frequently and taking a lighter view of life, you will find that life is much more enjoyable and fun. Here are three effective tips to help you get more laughter in your life:

both a
One of
kids rea
kids of
neighb
Become
Leagues
dren's e
and enj

TIP 1: FIND A COMIC STRIP TH
AND FOLLOW

Humor is very individual. What I
not, but the comics, or "funny pap
everybody. Read them thoroughly
you find particularly funny and lool

TIP 2: WATCH COMEDIES ON T
COMEDIES AT THE MO

With modern cable systems it is p
funny on television at virtually any
Find a show that you enjoy and wa
I am glad *Seinfeld* has gone into sy
night. If I do not have time to w
later.

My wife and I love to go t
good comedy. There is something
The more people in the theater, th
find yourself laughing. I have seen
I thought were absolutely hysteri
them at home on television or vi
what I thought was so funny abo
ambience and energy greatly inc
good laugh.

TIP 3: PLAY WI

My wife and I are truly blessed t
beautiful little girl, our Alexa (a.k

Chapter 5

Nutritional Factors

in Depression

There are a number of important nutritional factors to consider in the depressed individual. First of all, since the brain requires a constant supply of blood sugar, hypoglycemia must be avoided. As discussed in Chapter 3, hypoglycemia is a major cause of depression. In addition to glucose, the brain also requires a constant supply of other nutrients. It is a well-established fact that virtually any nutrient deficiency can result in impaired mental function. To function optimally the human brain requires virtually every known nutrient. Some nutrients are utilized in the transmission of information from nerve cell to nerve cell, others are involved in the manufacture of important brain compounds or perform vital roles in brain chemistry.

A deficiency of any single nutrient can alter brain function and lead to depression, anxiety, and other mental disorders. However, the role of nutrient deficiency is just the tip of the iceberg in regard to the role of nutrient effects on the brain and mood. According to Melvin Werbach, M.D., a faculty member at the UCLA School of Medicine and author of *Nutritional Influences on Mental Illness: A Sourcebook of Clinical Research*, "It is clear that nutrition can powerfully influence cognition, emotion, and behavior. It is also clear that the effects of classical nutritional deficiency diseases upon mental function constitute only a small part of a rapidly expanding list of interfaces between nutrition and the mind."

Table 5.1 Behavioral Effects of Some Vitamin Deficiencies

Deficient Vitamin	Behavioral Effects
Thiamine	Korsakoff's psychosis, mental depression, apathy, anxiety, irritability
Riboflavin	Depression, irritability
Niacin	Apathy, anxiety, depression, hyperirritability, mania, memory deficits, delirium, organic dementia, emotional lability
Biotin	Depression, extreme lassitude, somnolence
Pantothenic acid	Restlessness, irritability, depression, fatigue

Deficient Vitamin	Behavioral Effects
B$_6$	Depression, irritability, sensitivity to sound
Folic acid	Forgetfulness, insomnia, apathy, irritability, depression, psychosis, delirium, dementia
B$_{12}$	Psychotic states, depression, irritability, confusion, memory loss, hallucinations, delusions, paranoia
Vitamin C	Lassitude, hypochondriasis, depression, hysteria

Correcting an underlying nutritional deficiency can restore normal mental function and relieve depression. However, according to Dr. Werbach, the leading expert in the field of nutrition and mental function, "Even in the absence of laboratory validation of nutritional deficiencies, numerous studies utilizing rigorous scientific designs have demonstrated impressive benefits from nutritional supplementation."[1]

This chapter will outline dietary and nutritional supplement guidelines to ensure that the brain is constantly bathed in a nutrient-rich environment and has the necessary building blocks it needs to function optimally.

Dietary Guidelines

The dietary guidelines for depression are identical to the dietary guidelines for optimal health. It is now a well-established fact that certain dietary practices cause, while others prevent, a wide range of diseases. Quite simply, a health-promoting diet provides optimal levels of all known nutrients and low levels of food components that are detrimental to health, such as sugar, saturated fats, cholesterol, salt, and food additives. A health-promoting diet is rich in whole "natural" and unprocessed foods. It is especially high in plant foods, such as fruits, vegetables, grains, beans, seeds and nuts, as these foods not only contain valuable nutrients but additional compounds that have remarkable health-promoting properties. Here are seven steps to a health-promoting diet:

Step 1: Reduce your fat intake

Current recommendations are that total fat intake be less than 30 percent of calories, with less than 10 percent of calories coming from saturated fat, and that the intake of cholesterol be less than 300 mg daily. The easiest way to achieve these recommendations is to limit your intake of animal products and not to use butter, margarine, salad dressings, gravy, creamy sauces, or other high-fat foods.

Step 2: Eat five or more servings of vegetables and fruits

Fruits and vegetables are rich in fiber, vitamins, minerals, antioxidants, and dozens of recently discovered phytochemicals that protect our body cells from damage. A high intake of fruits and vegetables has been shown to help protect against aging, cancer, heart disease, and many other degenerative conditions. Despite the well-known health benefits of frequent fruit and vegetable intake, fewer than 10 percent of all Americans eat the recommended quantity of five or more servings daily.

Step 3: Limit your refined-sugar intake

Carbohydrates provide us with the energy we need for body functions. There are two groups of carbohydrates, simple and complex. Simple carbohydrates, or sugars, are quickly absorbed by the body for a ready source of energy. The assortment of natural simple sugars in plant foods has an advantage over sucrose (white sugar) and other refined sugars in that they are balanced by fiber and a wide range of nutrients that aid in their utilization. Problems with carbohydrates begin when they are refined and stripped of these nutrients. Virtually all of the vitamin content has been removed from white sugar, white breads and pastries, and many breakfast cereals. When high-sugar foods are eaten alone, the blood sugar level rises quickly, producing a strain on blood sugar control. Sources of refined sugar should be limited, especially if you suffer from hypoglycemia. Read food labels carefully for clues on sugar content. If the words *sucrose, glucose, maltose, lactose, fructose, corn syrup,* or *white grape juice concentrate* appear on the label, extra sugar has been added.

Step 4: Increase your fiber and complex carbohydrate intake

While refined carbohydrates should be restricted, the intake of high-fiber complex carbohydrates should be increased. Complex carbohydrates, or starches, are composed of many simple sugars (polysaccharides) joined together by chemical bonds. The body breaks these bonds, releasing the simple sugars gradually, which leads to better blood sugar control. More and more research is indicating that complex carbohydrates should form a major part of the diet. Vegetables, legumes, and whole grains are excellent sources of high-fiber complex carbohydrates. A high-fiber diet has been shown to protect against the development of many chronic degenerative diseases.

Step 5: Maintain protein intake at moderate levels

After water, protein is the next most plentiful component of our body. The body manufactures proteins to make up hair, muscles, nails, tendons, ligaments, and other body structures. Proteins also function as enzymes, hormones, and as important components of other cells, such as our genes. Adequate protein intake is essential to good health, but too much protein causes problems.

One of the key recommendations of the National Research Council's Committee on Diet and Health was that Americans need to reduce protein intake to moderate levels. Americans consume much more protein than is required. Excess protein intake has been linked to several chronic diseases including cancer, osteoporosis, kidney disease, and heart disease. Reducing protein intake is best done by reducing meat and dairy consumption. Limit your intake to no more than 4 to 6 ounces per day and choose fish or skinless poultry. When you do eat meat, choose lean cuts rather than fat-laden choices.

Step 6: Limit your salt intake

The balance of sodium to potassium is extremely important to human health. Too much sodium in the diet can lead to disruption of this balance. In our society only 5% of sodium intake comes from the natural ingredients in food. Prepared foods contribute 45% of our sodium intake, 45% is added in cooking, and another 5% is added as a condiment. Excessive consumption of dietary sodium chloride (table salt), coupled with diminished dietary potassium from fruits and vegetables, plays a major role in the development of cancer and cardiovascular disease (heart disease, high blood pressure, strokes, etc.). Conversely, a diet high in potassium and low in sodium is protective against these diseases, and, in the case of high blood pressure, can be therapeutic. To reduce your intake of sodium:

- Learn to enjoy the unsalted flavor of foods.
- Cook with only small amounts of salt and use flavor-enhancing herbs and "salt substitutes."
- Limit your intake of heavily salted foods, such as potato chips, pretzels, cheese, pickled foods, and cured meats.
- Read food labels carefully and avoid highly salted prepared or packaged foods.

Step 7: Take the time for menu planning

Most Americans do not take any time to think about menu planning. Instead they find themselves in a rush and often resort to eating out at a fast-food restaurant or skipping a meal. Both practices can have a negative effect on health. Take a few minutes each evening to plan out the next day's menu. Or, if you can do it, plan out a menu for the week. You'll more than recoup the time because you'll shop more efficiently and won't find yourself missing some ingredient for the night's meal. In addition, you'll likely save money since less browsing makes it easier to avoid impulse buys. Here are some healthful menu suggestions:

BREAKFAST

Time and again, studies have shown that people who eat breakfast weigh less, have more energy, and enjoy better health. Healthy breakfast choices include whole grain cereals, muffins, and breads along with fresh whole fruit or fresh fruit juice. Cereals, both hot and cold, preferably from whole grains, may be the best choices. Not only do the complex carbohydrates in the grains provide sustained energy, but an evaluation of data from the National Health and Nutrition Examination Survey II (a national survey of the nutritional and health practices of Americans) showed that serum cholesterol levels were lowest among adults eating whole grain cereal for breakfast.[2] Although those individuals who consumed other breakfast foods had higher blood cholesterol levels, levels were highest among those who typically skipped breakfast.

LUNCH

Lunch is a great time to enjoy a healthful bowl of soup, a large salad, and some whole-grain bread. Due to their ability to improve blood sugar regulation, bean soups and other legume dishes are especially good lunch selections for people with diabetes and blood sugar problems. Beans and legumes are an excellent source of protein and fiber, yet low in fat and calories.

SNACKS

The best snacks are a handful of nuts or seeds, and some fresh fruit and vegetables (including fresh fruit and vegetable juice).

DINNER

For dinner the healthiest meals contain a fresh vegetable salad, a cooked vegetable side dish or bowl of soup, some whole grains, and legumes. The whole grains may be provided in bread, pasta, as a side dish, or as part of the recipe for an entrée. The legumes can be utilized in soups, salads, and entrées.

Although a mixed, varied diet rich in whole grains, vegetables, and legumes can provide optimal levels of protein, many people like to eat meat. The important thing is not to overconsume animal products. Again, limit your intake to no more than 4 to 6 ounces per day and choose fish or skinless poultry. When you do eat red meat, opt for lean cuts rather than fat-laden choices.

Recommendations for
Nutritional Supplementation

Many Americans consume a diet inadequate in nutritional value yet not to a point where obvious deficiencies are apparent. The term *subclinical,* or marginal, deficiency is often used to describe this concept. A subclinical deficiency indicates a deficiency of a particular vitamin or mineral that is not severe enough to produce a classic deficiency sign or symptom. Complicating the matter is the fact that in many instances the only clue of a subclinical nutrient deficiency may be fatigue, lethargy, difficulty in concentration, a lack of well-being, or some other vague symptom. Diagnosis of subclinical deficiencies is an extremely difficult process that involves detailed dietary or laboratory analysis.

Is there evidence to support the contention that subclinical vitamin and mineral deficiencies exist? Definitely yes. During recent years the U.S. government has sponsored a number of comprehensive studies (HANES I and II, Ten State Nutrition Survey, USDA nationwide food consumption studies, etc.) to determine the nutritional status of the population. These studies have revealed that marginal nutrient deficiencies exist in a substantial portion of the U.S. population (approximately 50 percent) and that for some selected nutrients in certain age groups more than 80 percent of the group consumed less than the RDA.[3]

These studies indicate that the chances of consuming a

diet meeting the recommended dietary allowance (RDA) for all nutrients is extremely unlikely for most Americans. In other words while it is theoretically possible that a healthy individual can get all the nutrition he or she needs from foods, the fact is that most Americans do not even come close to meeting all their nutritional needs through diet alone. In an effort to increase their intake of essential nutrients, many Americans look to vitamin and mineral supplements.

Is the RDA Enough?

Recommended Dietary Allowances (RDAs) for vitamins and minerals have been prepared by the Food and Nutrition Board of the National Research Council since 1941.[4] These guidelines were originally developed to reduce the rates of severe nutritional deficiency diseases such as scurvy (deficiency of vitamin C), pellagra (deficiency of niacin), and beri-beri (deficiency of vitamin B_1). Another critical point is that the RDAs were designed to serve as the basis for evaluating the adequacy of diets of groups of people, not individuals. Individuals simply vary too widely in their nutritional requirements. As stated by the Food and Nutrition Board, "Individuals with special nutritional needs are not covered by the RDAs."

A tremendous amount of scientific research indicates that the "optimal" level for many nutrients, especially the so-called antioxidant nutrients such as vitamins C and E, beta-carotene, and selenium, may be much higher than their current RDA. The RDAs focus only on the prevention of nutritional deficiencies in population groups, they do not define "optimal" intake for an individual.

Another factor the RDAs do not adequately take into consideration are environmental and lifestyle factors, which can destroy vitamins and bind minerals. For example, even the Food and Nutrition Board acknowledges that smokers require at least twice as much vitamin C compared with non-smokers.[4] But what about other nutrients and smoking? And what about the effects of alcohol consumption, food additives, heavy metals (lead, mercury, etc.), carbon monoxide, and other chemicals associated with our modern society that are known to interfere with nutrient function? Dealing with hazards of modern living may be another reason why many people take supplements.

While the RDAs have done a good job at defining nutrient intake levels to prevent nutritional deficiencies, there is still much to be learned regarding the optimum intake of nutrients.

Take a High-Potency Multiple Vitamin and Mineral Formula

A high-potency multiple provides a good nutritional foundation upon which to build. When selecting a multiple vitamin and mineral formula it is important to make sure that it provides the full range of vitamins and minerals at high-potency levels. Here is the desirable supplementation range

for the individual vitamins and minerals in a high-potency
multiple vitamin and mineral formula; the product should
provide a daily dosage of the following nutrients:

Vitamins

Vitamin A (retinol)	5,000–10,000 IU
Vitamin A (from beta-carotene)	10,000–25,000 IU
Vitamin D	100–400 IU
Vitamin E (d-alpha tocopherol)	200–400 IU
Vitamin K (phytonadione)	60–900 mcg
Vitamin C (ascorbic acid)	500–1,000 mg
Vitamin B_1 (thiamine)	10–90 mg
Vitamin B_2 (riboflavin)	10–90 mg
Niacin	10–90 mg
Niacinamide	10–30 mg
Vitamin B_6 (pyridoxine)	25–100 mg
Biotin	100–300 mcg
Pantothenic acid	25–100 mg
Folic acid	400–1,000 mcg
Vitamin B_{12}	400–1,000 mcg
Choline	150–500 mg
Inositol	150–500 mg

Minerals

Boron	1–2 mg
Calcium	250–750 mg
Chromium	200–400 mcg
Copper	1–2 mg
Iodine	50–150 mcg

Minerals (*cont.*)

Iron	15–30 mg
Magnesium	250–750 mg
Manganese	10–15 mg
Molybdenum	10–25 mcg
Potassium	200–500 mg
Selenium	100–200 mcg
Silica	200–1,000 mcg
Vanadium	50–100 mcg
Zinc	15–30 mg

Individual Nutrients and Depression

Deficiencies of a number of specific nutrients are quite common in depressed individuals. The most common deficiencies are folic acid, vitamin B_{12}, and vitamin B_6. The significance of these deficiencies is discussed below.

FOLIC ACID AND VITAMIN B_{12}

Folic acid and vitamin B_{12} function together in many biochemical processes. Folic acid deficiency is the most common nutrient deficiency in the world. In studies of depressed patients as many as 31 to 35 percent have been shown to be deficient in folic acid.[5] In elderly patients this percentage may be even higher, as one study found that among elderly patients admitted to a psychiatric ward the number of patients with folic acid deficiency has been reported to range from 35 to 92.6%.[6] Depression is the most common symptom of a folic acid deficiency. Vitamin B_{12} deficiency is less common than that of folic acid deficiency, but it can also cause depression, especially in the elderly.[7] Correcting the folic acid and/or vitamin B_{12} deficiency results in a dramatic improvement in mood.[8]

Folic acid, vitamin B_{12}, and a form of the amino acid methionine known as SAM (S-adenosyl-methionine) function as "methyl donors." They carry and donate methyl molecules to important brain compounds including neurotransmitters. SAM is the major methyl donor in the body. The antidepressant effects of folic acid appear to be a result of raising brain SAM content. SAM is discussed in greater detail in Chapter 9.

One of the key brain compounds dependent upon methylation is tetrahydrobiopterin (BH4). This compound functions as an essential coenzyme in the activation of enzymes that manufacture monoamine neurotransmitters such as serotonin and dopamine from their corresponding amino acids. Patients with recurrent depression have been shown to have reduced BH4 synthesis, probably as a result of low SAM levels. BH4 supplementation has been shown to produce dramatic results in these patients.[8] Unfortunately BH4 is not currently available commercially. However, since BH4 synthesis is stimulated by folic acid, vitamin B_{12}, and vitamin C, it is possible that increasing these vitamin levels in the brain may stimulate BH4 formation and the synthesis of monoamines such as serotonin.[9]

There is evidence to support the contention that supplementing the diet with folic acid, vitamin C, and vitamin B_{12} can increase BH4 levels. In addition the folic acid supplementation and the promotion of methylation reactions has been shown to increase the serotonin content.[10] The serotonin-elevating effects are undoubtedly responsible for much of the antidepressive effects of folic acid and vitamin B_{12}. Typically the dosages used in the clinical studies where folic acid has been used as an antidepressant have been very high: 15 mg to 50 mg. Dosages of folate this high require a doctor's prescription. High-dose folic acid therapy is safe (except in patients with epilepsy) and has been shown to be as effective as antidepressant drugs.[11] However, there are other natural measures described in this book that yield even better results (e.g., St. John's wort extract and SAM).

A dosage of 800 mcg of folic acid and 800 mcg of vitamin B_{12} should be sufficient in most circumstances to prevent deficiencies. Folic acid supplementation should always be accompanied by vitamin B_{12} supplementation to prevent folic acid from masking a vitamin B_{12} deficiency.

VITAMIN B_6

Vitamin B_6 levels are typically quite low in depressed patients, especially women taking birth control pills or Premarin.[12] Considering the many functions of vitamin B_6 in the brain, including the fact that vitamin B_6 is absolutely essential in the manufacture of all monoamines, it is likely that many of the millions of people who are taking Prozac may be suffering depression simply as a result of low vitamin B_6. Patients with low B_6 status usually respond very well to supplementation. The typical effective dosage is 50 mg to 100 mg.

FLAXSEED OIL

A recommendation to supplement your diet with one table-spoon of flaxseed oil may have you confused. However, this recommendation makes perfectly good sense. While it is true Americans should not consume more than 30 percent of daily calories as fats, a lack of the dietary essential fatty acids, especially the omega-3 fatty acids, has been suggested to play a significant role in the development of many chronic degenerative diseases, such as heart disease, cancer, and stroke.[13]

It is estimated by many experts that approximately 80 percent of our population consumes an insufficient quantity of essential fatty acids. This dietary insufficiency presents a serious health threat to Americans. In addition to providing the body with energy, the essential fatty acids, linoleic and linolenic acid, provided by plant foods function in our bodies as components of nerve cells, cellular membranes, and hormonelike substances known as prostaglandins. Prostaglandins and the essential fatty acids are important for the regulation of a host of bodily functions. They

- Maintain the fluidity of cellular membranes
- Manufacture hormones
- Regulate pressure in the eye, joints, and blood vessels
- Regulate response to pain, inflammation, and swelling
- Mediate immune response

- Regulate bodily secretions and their viscosity
- Dilate and constrict blood vessels
- Regulate collateral circulation
- Direct endocrine hormones to their target cells
- Regulate smooth muscle and autonomic reflexes
- Are primary constituents of cellular membranes
- Regulate the rate at which cells divide (mitosis)
- Regulate the flow of substances into and out of the cells
- Are important for the transport of oxygen from the red blood cell to the bodily tissues
- Regulate kidney function and fluid balance
- Are important in keeping saturated fats mobile in the bloodstream
- Prevent blood cells from clumping together (conglomeration) (the cause of atherosclerotic plaque and blood clots, a cause of stroke)
- Mediate the release of pro-inflammatory substances from cells that may trigger allergic conditions
- Regulate nerve transmission
- Are the primary energy source for the heart muscle

As well as playing a critical role in normal physiology, essential fatty acids are being shown to actually be protective and therapeutic against heart disease, cancer, autoimmune diseases such as multiple sclerosis and rheumatoid arthritis, many skin diseases, and many others. Over sixty health conditions have now been shown to benefit from essential fatty acid supplementation.

Major health conditions benefited by essential fatty acid supplementation include the following:

Acne	High blood pressure
AIDS	Hyperactivity
Allergies	Infant nutrition
Alzheimer's	Lupus
Arthritis	Malnutrition
Atherosclerosis	Menopause
Brain development	Mental illness
Breast cysts	Multiple sclerosis
Breast pain	Postangioplasty
Cancer	Postcoronary bypass
Cystic fibrosis	Postviral fatigue
Dermatitis	Pregnancy
Dry skin	Psoriasis
Eczema	Rheumatoid arthritis

The Cause of the Essential Fatty Acid Deficiency

What has caused this deficiency of essential fatty acids (EFA)? Mass commercial refinement of fats and oils and foods containing them has effectively eliminated the essential fatty acids from our food chain. In addition there has been a tremendous increase in the amount of unnatural fats and oils added to the diet in the form of trans-fatty acids and partially hydrogenated oils. In 1909 Americans consumed about 125 g of fat per day.

Today the consumption is closer to 175 g per day, an increase of some 40 percent, or about fifty extra pounds, per year. What remains untold is that there has actually been a reduced ingestion of natural, unadulterated essential fatty acids. Instead Americans have drastically increased the ingestion of refined and adulterated fats and oils. These refined and processed compounds actually inhibit the body's ability to utilize the essential fatty acids that are consumed.

The signs and symptoms of essential fatty acid deficiency may be either overt or chronically nagging, ranging from mild fatigue to fatal heart attack. Most orthodox health care practitioners may never make the association between a health symptom and essential fatty acid deficiency, therefore the underlying cause of illness will ultimately continue to manifest. Most physicians are not trained in nutrition to begin with, and the laboratory analysis to measure essential fatty acid deficiency is not widely available or appreciated. In addition the symptoms of essential fatty acid deficiency are not as obvious as with many other nutrient deficiencies. Regardless, the consequences are far more deadly in this day and age. Even if an essential fatty acid deficiency were recognized, few orthodox clinicians would know how to treat it.

In general, a deficiency of essential fatty acids can be so vague and broad that symptoms typically are written off as one of a myriad of other causes. Here are some signs and symptoms typical, but not exclusive, to EFA deficiency:

- Depression
- Fatigue, malaise, lack of energy

- Forgetfulness
- Lack of endurance
- Lack of motivation
- Dry skin
- Cracked nails
- Dry, lifeless hair
- Dry mucous membranes, tear ducts, mouth, vagina
- Maldigestion, gas, bloating
- Constipation
- Immune weakness
- Frequent colds and sickness
- Aching, sore joints
- Angina, chest pain
- High blood pressure
- History of cardiovascular disease
- Arthritis

Organic, unrefined flaxseed oil is considered by many to be the answer to restoring the proper level of essential fatty acids. Flaxseed oil is unique because it contains both essential fatty acids: alpha linolenic (an omega-3 fatty acid) and linoleic acid (an omega-6 fatty acid) in appreciable amounts. Flaxseed oil is the world's richest source of omega-3 fatty acids. At a whopping 58 percent by weight, it contains over two times the amount of omega-3 fatty acids as fish oils. Omega-3 fatty acids have been extensively studied for their beneficial effects in relation to the following:

High cholesterol levels

Stroke and heart attack

Angina (heart pain)

High blood pressure

Arthritis

Multiple sclerosis

Psoriasis, eczema, and other inflammatory skin
    disorders

Inhibiting cancer formation and metastasis

Omega-3 Fatty Acids and Depression

An insufficiency of omega-3 oils is also linked to depression.[14]
All cells throughout the human body are enveloped by membranes composed chiefly of essential fatty acids in the form of
phospholipids. Phospholipids play a major role in determining
the integrity and fluidity of cell membranes. What determines
the type of phospholipid in the cell membrane is the type of
fat consumed. Although we can ingest preformed phospholipids such as lecithin or phosphatidylcholine and phosphatidylserine (discussed further on pages 165–166), most of these
phospholipids are broken down into glycerol, free fatty acids,
and the phosphate group rather than being incorporated in-
tact into cellular membranes.

A phospholipid composed of a saturated fat or trans-fatty
acid differs considerably in structure from a phospholipid
composed of an essential fatty acid. In addition there are differences between the structure of an omega-3 oil composed

membrane and an omega-6 composed membrane. Membranes composed of omega-3 oils are more fluid.

While it is thought the cell is programmed to selectively incorporate the different fatty acids it needs to maintain optimal function, because of the lack of essential fatty acids (particularly the omega-3 oils) in the standard American diet, in actuality what becomes incorporated into the cell membranes is determined primarily by diet. A diet composed of largely saturated fat, animal fatty acids (e.g., arachidonic acid), cholesterol, and trans-fatty acids is going to lead to membranes that are much less fluid in nature than the membranes of an individual consuming optimum levels of both essential fatty acids.

A relative deficiency of essential fatty acids in cellular membranes makes it virtually impossible for the cell membrane to perform its vital function. The basic function of the cell membrane is to serve as a selective barrier that regulates the passage of certain materials in and out of the cell. When there is a disturbance of structure or function of the cell membrane, there is a tremendous disruption of homeostasis. This term, *homeostasis,* refers to the maintenance of static, or constant, conditions in the internal environment of the cell and, on a larger scale, the human body as a whole. In other words, with a disturbance in cellular membrane structure or function, there is disruption of virtually all cellular processes.

Because the brain is the richest source of phospholipids in the human body and proper nerve cell function is critically dependent on proper membrane fluidity, it only makes sense that alterations in membrane fluidity could dramatically impact behavior, mood, and mental function. In addition, studies have shown that the biophysical properties, including fluidity, of brain cell membranes directly influences neurotransmitter synthesis, signal transmission, uptake of serotonin and other neurotransmitters, neurotransmitter binding, and the activity of monoamine oxidase. All of these factors have been implicated in depression and other psychological disturbances.

Researchers have concluded that omega-3 fatty acids may reduce the development of depression just as they reduce the development of coronary artery disease.[14] This conclusion was based on several factors:

- Recent studies have suggested that lowering plasma cholesterol by diet and medications increases suicide, homicide, and depression.
- The quantity and type of dietary fats consumed influences serum lipids and alters the biophysical and biochemical properties of cell membranes.
- Dietary advice to lower cholesterol levels tends to increase the ratio of omega-6 to omega-3 and decreases the level of the important omega-3 fatty acid, docosahexanoic acid.
- Epidemiological studies in various countries and the United States have indicated that decreased consumption of omega-3 fatty acids correlates with increasing rates of depression.
- There is also a consistent association between depression and coronary artery disease.

Hopefully now that these associations have been stated and supported in the medical literature, it will inspire other researchers to examine the therapeutic potential of omega-3 fatty acids in depression and other disturbed psychological states. In the meantime, supplementing the diet with one tablespoon of a high-quality flaxseed oil makes great sense.

The brand of flaxseed oil that I recommend is Barlean's. It is the highest quality and best-tasting brand. Barlean's Flax Oil can be found in most health food stores. To find a store in your area, call 1-800-445-FLAX (3529).

Final Comments

Proper mental function requires a constant supply of high nutrition to the brain. The quality of the food and nutritional supplements you ingest plays a big role in the quality of your mental function and mood. Feed your brain the nutrition it needs by following the seven steps to a healthful diet given in this chapter, taking a high-potency multiple vitamin and mineral formula and taking one tablespoon of a high-quality flaxseed oil product. These recommendations provide the nutritional foundation upon which to build.

Chapter 6

St. John's Wort Extract

A n extract of St. John's wort standardized to contain 0.3 percent hypericin is perhaps the most effective natural antidepressant currently available. St. John's wort is a shrubby perennial plant with numerous bright yellow flowers. It is commonly found in dry, rocky soils, fields, and sunny places. St. John's wort is native to many parts of the world including Europe and the United States. It grows especially well in northern California and southern Oregon.

St. John's wort has a long history of folk use. Many people from the time of the ancient Greeks through the Middle Ages believed St. John's wort to have magical powers. Its Latin name, *Hypericum perforatum,* is derived from Greek— *Hyper* ("over") *eikon* ("image," in the sense of a ghost)—and signifies the belief that the plant exerted magical properties over ghosts. The common name, St. John's wort, also has its origins in folk traditions. Two stories predominate. One story states that the red spots are symbolic of the blood of St. John and first appeared on the leaves of the plant on the anniversary of the saint's beheading. Another story comes from a common medieval belief that if one slept with a piece of the plant under his or her pillow on St. John's Eve, the saint would appear in a dream, give his blessing, and prevent one from dying during the following year.

St. John's wort has historically been used as a nerve tonic. Presumably this use also extended to the treatment of depression and anxiety.

St. John's Wort Extract in Germany

The extract of St. John's wort, standardized to contain 0.3 percent hypericin, is quickly becoming a popular prescription for depression in Germany. Herbal products there can be marketed with drug claims if they have been proven to be safe and effective. Actually the legal requirements for herbal medicines are identical to those of all other drugs. Whether the herbal product is available by prescription or over the counter is based upon its application and safety of use. Herbal products sold in pharmacies are reimbursed by insurance if they are prescribed by a physician.

The proof required by a manufacturer in Germany to illustrate safety and effectiveness for an herbal product is far less than the proof required by the Food and Drug Administration for drugs in the United States. In Germany a special commission (Commission E) developed a series of two hundred monographs on herbal products similar to the over-the-counter monographs in the United States. An herbal product is viewed as safe and effective if a manufacturer meets the quality requirements of the monograph or produces additional evidence of safety and effectiveness that can include data from existing literature, anecdotal information from practicing physicians, as well as limited clinical studies.

In the United States, because a plant cannot be patented, drug companies screen plants for biological activity and then the so-called active constituents (compounds) are isolated. If the compound is powerful enough, the drug company will begin the process to procure FDA approval. Because of the expense and lack of patent protection, very little research has been done during this century on whole plants or crude plant extracts as medicinal agents per se by the large American pharmaceutical firms. In contrast, European policies have made it economically feasible for companies to research and develop herbs as medicines. St. John's wort extract is just one example of a European phytopharmaceutical (plant-derived drug). Two other herbal antidepressants, Ginkgo biloba extract and kava extract, will be discussed in their own chapters. In the United States, consumers can find herbal extracts in health food stores and some pharmacies that are identical to the phytopharmaceuticals in use in Europe. In the United States manufacturers of these extracts are prohibited from making any therapeutic claims for their products.

The official German Commission E monograph for St. John's wort lists psychovegetative disturbance, depressive states, fear and nervous disturbances as clinical indications for the extract.

St. John's Wort Extract as an Antidepressant

St. John's wort extract is the most thoroughly researched natural antidepressant. A total of 1,592 patients have been studied in twenty-five double-blind controlled studies (fifteen compared with placebo, ten compared with antidepressant drugs including five studies comparing St. John's wort with tricyclics: two versus imipramine; two versus amitriptyline; and one versus desipramine.)[1]

In these studies, St. John's wort extract was shown to produce improvements in many psychological symptoms including depression, anxiety, apathy, sleep disturbances, insomnia, anorexia, and feelings of worthlessness. Even more impressive is that St. John's wort extract was able to achieve these benefits without producing a side effect. Before examining these head-to-head studies, let's examine the most recent double-blind placebo-controlled study.

In the study, 105 patients with different types of mild to moderate depressions were given either 300 mg of the St. John's wort extract standardized to contain 0.3% hypericin or an identical-looking placebo three times daily for four weeks.[2] The effectiveness of treatment was judged after two and four weeks according to the Hamilton Depression Scale (HAMD), the standard measure to assess an antidepressant's effectiveness. Here are the results:

	St. John's Wort	Placebo
Baseline	15.81	15.83
Week 2	9.64	12.28
Week 4	7.17	11.30

Using the criteria of a decrease in the HAMD of greater than 50%, or achieving a value less than ten as identification of responders, twenty-eight out of forty-two patients (67%) in the St. John's wort group responded compared with only thirteen of forty-seven patients (27.7%) in the placebo group. The results of this study are consistent with other well-designed studies comparing St. John's wort with placebo.[3]

The studies comparing St. John's wort with tricyclic antidepressants have also demonstrated a therapeutic advantage for St. John's wort.[1] For example in one double-blind study of 135 depressive patients given either St. John's wort extract or imipramine, significant advantages were shown with the St. John's wort in the main assessment criteria of three commonly used evaluation tools for antidepressant activity—HAMD, von Zerssen Depressive Scale (D-S), and Clinical Global Impressions (CGI).[4] The most significant improvements were noted in HAMD and D-S:

	St. Johns Wort	Imipramine
Hamilton Depression Scale		
Initial measurement	20.2	19.4
Week 6	8.8	10.7
Depression Scale (von Zerssen)		
Initial measurement	39.6	39
Week 6	27.2	29.2

The main advantage in other studies with the St. John's wort extract versus antidepressant drugs was not so much a difference in therapeutic outcome but rather a significant advantage in terms of side effects and patient tolerance in the St. John's wort group. For example, in a study of 102 patients there were slightly better results obtained with maprotiline (a tetracyclic) in the HAMD, D-S, and CGI, but when side effects and patient tolerance are added to the equation, St. John's wort comes out on top.[5] Maprotiline treatment resulted in the typical side effects with tricyclics, for example, tiredness, mouth dryness, and heart complaints.

One of the most interesting comparative studies was a double-blind study where St. John's wort extract was compared with maprotiline in twenty-four healthy volunteers by measuring resting brain wave (EEG) tracings and mental activity (visual and acoustic evoked potentials).[6] Interpretation of the differences in reactions indicated that unlike maprotiline, which interferes with mental function, St. John's wort actually improves memory and other mental activities.

St. John's wort has also been shown to improve sleep quality and well-being in healthy elderly subjects.[7] With antidepressant drugs, particularly tricyclic antidepressants and MAO inhibitors, REM (rapid eye movement) sleep is reduced. It is during REM that we dream. St. John's wort did not interfere with REM sleep like other antidepressants and was shown to increase the intensity of deep sleep during the total sleeping period, as demonstrated by brain wave studies. While St. John's wort improved sleep quality, it did not act as a sedative (i.e., it did not reduce sleep onset), nor did it change total sleep duration.

How Does St. John's Wort Extract Work?

St. John's wort extract is thought to alter brain chemistry in a favorable manner. Specifically, hypericin and other components (particularly flavonoids) of St. John's wort have been shown to inhibit the breakdown of several neurotransmitters including serotonin.[8] As a result of this inhibition there is an increase in the level of nerve impulse transmitters within the brain that maintain normal mood and emotional stability. However, the antidepressive effect of St. John's wort extract cannot be explained totally in terms of inhibiting the breakdown of monoamines. Other mechanisms will likely be discovered. For example, St. John's wort also appears to improve

the signal produced by serotonin after it binds to its receptor on brain cells.

One of the first human studies with St. John's wort extract measured the change in urinary metabolites of noradrenaline and dopamine in six depressed women, aged fifty-five to sixty-five, after taking a standardized extract of St. John's wort extract (0.14% hypericin content).[9] Researchers found a significant increase in the metabolite 3-methoxy-4-hydroxyphenylglycol, a marker commonly used to evaluate the efficacy of antidepressant therapy.

In addition to human studies, extracts of St. John's wort have also been tested in various animal models designed to better understand its antidepressant effects. In these studies St. John's wort extract was found to enhance the exploratory activity of mice in a foreign environment; extend the sleeping time after the animals were given a narcotic; antagonize the effects of reserpine, a drug that depletes the brain of important neurotransmitters; and decrease aggressive behavior in socially isolated male mice.[1] These activities are consistent with the expected effects of antidepressant compounds.

Safety Issues

St. John's wort extract is virtually free of side effects at the standard dosage of 300 mg three times daily. No significant side effects have been reported in the numerous double-blind studies, but perhaps the best demonstration of the excellent safety record of St. John's wort extract is a large-scale study involving 3,250 patients conducted in Germany.[10] Results were analyzed by means of a patient questionnaire. Pooled data indicated that symptoms of depression were reduced in frequency and intensity by approximately 50%. The frequency of undesired side effects was reported in 79 patients (2.43%), and 48 (1.45%) discontinued therapy. The most frequently noted side effects were gastrointestinal irritation (0.55%), allergic reactions (0.52%), fatigue (0.4%), and restlessness (0.26%).

The frequency and severity of side effects with St. John's wort extract are clinically insignificant, especially when compared with the well-known side effects of tricyclics and other antidepressants.

Dosage

To get the same results noted in the many studies with St. John's wort, it is absolutely essential to utilize products identical to those used in the studies at the proper dosage. The St. John's wort extract must be standardized to contain 0.3% hypericin and be taken at the dosage of 300 mg three times daily.

Standardized extracts (also referred to as guaranteed potency extracts) refer to an extract guaranteed to contain a "standardized" level of active compounds. In the case of St. John's wort, the extract is standardized to contain 0.3% hypericin. Standardized extracts are produced according to strict quality-control standards and good manufacturing practices. They provide the greatest benefit because they state the level of active compounds and you are thus assured of quality and an accurate dosage.

Final Comments

St. John's wort extract offers a significant advantage over antidepressant drugs such as Prozac—safety. While St. John's wort is quite appropriate for use in cases of mild to moderate depression, it must be pointed out that St. John's wort is not yet suitable in the treatment of serious depressions (i.e., depressions associated with psychotic symptoms and/or depressions with serious risk of suicide).

Chapter 7

Kava Extract

Kava (*Piper methysticum*), a member of the pepper family, is one of the most fascinating of medicinal plants. For medicinal purposes it is the knotty, thick, pithy, and sometimes tuberous rootstock that is used. Native to the South Pacific, a beverage (also called kava) made from the rootstock of the plant has been used for centuries in ceremonies and celebrations because of its calming effect and ability to promote sociability. The kava beverage is still used today by inhabitants of the island communities of the Pacific including Micronesia, Melanesia, and Polynesia. It is thought that the frequent consumption of kava is partially why these people are referred to as the happiest and friendliest in the world.

The Kava Ceremony

Traditionally kava was only consumed during ceremonies. The ceremonies ranged from the full ceremonial enacted on every formal occasion to the kava circle common for less-formal social gatherings.[1] The first thing to do with any kava ceremony was the preparation of the beverage. A description of the classic process was given in 1777 by George Forster, a young naturalist on Captain James Cook's second Pacific voyage:

> [Kava] is made in the most disgustful manner that can be imagined, from the juice contained in the roots of a species of pepper-tree. This root is cut small, and the pieces chewed by several people, who spit the macerated mass into a bowl, where some water (milk) of coconuts is poured upon it. They then strain it through a quantity of fibres of coconuts, squeezing the chips, till all their juices mix with the coconut-milk; and the whole liquor is decanted into another bowl. They swallow this nauseous stuff as fast as possible; and some old topers value themselves on being able to empty a great number of bowls.

I assure you that the kava extract that will be described below is not produced via this traditional method of preparation. In fact, because the traditional method of preparing kava beverage was so disgusting to colonial governments and missionaries, they made it illegal for the natives to prepare it that way and forced them to prepare the beverage by grinding or grating the rootstock.

Kava induces a pleasant sense of tranquillity and sociability after it is consumed. Over the years many scientists have consumed kava in an attempt to describe its effects in more scientific terms. One of the first such descriptions of kava was offered by the noted pharmacologist Louis Lewin in 1886. Lewin must have enjoyed studying kava, because what became his classic description of kava's effects was written in 1927, over forty years after his initial investigation. Here is Lewin's classic description:

> When the mixture is not too strong, the subject attains a state of happy unconcern, well-being and contentment, free of physical or psychological excitement. At the beginning conversation comes in a gentle, easy flow and hearing and sight are honed, becoming able to perceive subtle shades of sound and vision. Kava soothes temperaments. The drinker never becomes angry, unpleasant, quarrelsome or noisy, as happens with alcohol. Both natives and whites consider kava as a means of easing moral discomfort. The drinker remains master of his conscious and his reason. When consumption is excessive, however, the limbs become tired, the muscles seem no longer to respond to the orders and control of the mind, walking becomes slow and unsteady and the drinker looks partially inebriated. He feels the need to

lie down. . . . He is overcome by somnolence and finally drifts off to sleep.[1]

A more recent description is provided by researcher R. J. Gregory, who writes from his own experience:

> Kava seizes one's mind. This is not a literal seizure, but something does change in the processes by which information enters, is retrieved, or leads to actions as a result. Thinking is certainly affected by the kava experience, but not in the same ways as are found from caffeine, nicotine, alcohol, or marijuana. I would personally characterize the changes I experienced as going from lineal processing of information to a greater sense of "being" and contentment with being. Memory seemed to be enhanced, whereas restriction of data inputs was strongly desired, especially with regard to disturbances of light, movements, noise and so on. Peace and quiet were very important to maintain the inner sense of serenity. My senses seemed to be unusually sharpened, so that even whispers seemed to be loud while loud noises were extremely unpleasant.[1]

The difference between the effect noted by these pharmacologists consuming kava beverage and the effect of the kava extract that will be described in this chapter is a matter of dosage. During the traditional kava ceremony an individual will usually ingest much higher amounts of kava components compared with the levels commonly used in the treatment of depression and anxiety. The kava extract could produce the same type of effects as kava beverage if taken at high levels (not recommended).

Kava Extracts in Anxiety and Depression

Like St. John's wort, kava extracts are gaining in popularity in Europe in the treatment of anxiety and depression. Several European countries (e.g., Germany, United Kingdom, Switzerland, and Austria) have approved kava preparations in the treatment of nervous anxiety, insomnia, and restlessness on the basis of detailed pharmacological data and favorable clinical studies. These approved kava preparations are extracts standardized for kavalactone content (usually 30 to 70 percent).

The kavalactones were deemed the active compounds in kava based on detailed scientific investigations over the past 110 years. However, although the kavalactones are the primary active components, other components appear to possess activity as well. Studies have shown that the relaxing and antianxiety effects of a crude kava preparation were more pronounced than those of the isolated kavalactones.[2] Studies have also shown that kavalactones are more rapidly absorbed when given in the kava extract rather than the isolated kavalactones. For example in one study the absorption of the kavalactones was shown to be three to five times higher from the extract compared with an equal amount of isolated kavalactones.[2] A study in animals demonstrated another impressive advantage—the brain uptake of kavalactones from a kava extract is two to twenty times higher than that achieved with isolated kavalactones.[3] Because the kavalactone content in crude preparations can vary between 3 and 20 percent, it is essential, when medicinal effects are desired, to utilize extracts standardized for kavalactone content. These standardized extracts provide the synergistic benefits along with a consistent therapeutic response because of the guaranteed level of kavalactones. The majority of the studies with standardized kava extracts have featured a special kava extract standardized to contain 70 percent kavalactones. However, this high percentage of kavalactones may be sacrificing some of the other constituents that may contribute to the pharmacology of kava.[4] Extracts standardized to contain 30 percent kavalactones may prove to be more effective than the 70 percent extract.

Before scientists knew of the benefits of using kava extracts standardized for kavalactone content, they studied the effect of isolated kavalactones in anxiety and depression. These studies demonstrated that isolated kavalactones were quite effective in relieving anxiety and depression. For example, in one double-blind placebo-controlled study eighty-four patients with anxiety symptoms were either given D,L-kavain, a purified kavalactone, at a dose of 400 mg per day or a placebo. The group receiving the purified kavalactone demonstrated improvements in anxiety symptoms and memory.[5] In another double-blind study thirty-eight patients were given either D,L-kavain or oxazepam, a drug similar to Valium (diazepam), for four weeks.[6] Both groups demonstrated improvements in two different anxiety scores (Anxiety

Status Inventory and the Self-Rating Anxiety Scale), however, while oxazepam and similar drugs are associated with being addictive, as well as possessing side effects, kavain was nonaddictive and was free of side effects.

More recent studies have utilized standardized kava extracts. For example, in one double-blind study fifty-eight patients suffering from anxiety were assigned to receive either 100 mg of the kava extract containing 70 percent kavalactones or a placebo three times daily for four weeks.[7] The group taking the kava extract exhibited significant improvements in several standard psychological assessments including the Hamilton Anxiety Scale. Symptoms of anxiety, such as feelings of nervousness, and somatic complaints, such as heart palpitations, chest pains, headache, dizziness, and feelings of gastric irritation, were either totally eliminated or greatly reduced. What is even more phenomenal than the excellent results that were obtained was the fact that they were obtained without side effects.

One group of patients who appear to respond extremely well to kava extract are women going through menopause— a time often associated with increased nervousness and anxiety. In a double-blind study forty menopausal women with menopause-related symptoms were given either 100 mg of the kava extract standardized to contain 70 percent kavalactones or a placebo three times daily for eight weeks.[8] The beneficial effects of the kava extract were almost immediate, as after one week there was a significant improvement in scores on the Hamilton Anxiety Scale in the group receiving the kava extract. As the trial continued, the scores continued to improve in the kava group. In addition to improvement in symptoms of stress and anxiety, the group receiving kava also noted improvements in feelings of well-being, mood, and menopausal symptoms including hot flashes. Again, these positive effects were gained without side effects.

One of the major drawbacks of benzodiazepines, besides their addictiveness, is that they impair mental function. That is the reason for the warning not to drive or operate heavy equipment while on these drugs. In contrast, according to results of studies in humans and animals, kava does not impair mental function. Instead it actually enhances it.[9]

In one study, twelve healthy volunteers were tested in a double-blind crossover manner to assess the effects of oxazepam (a benzodiazepine), the extract of kava standardized at 70 percent kavalactones (200 mg three times daily for five days), and a placebo on behavior and brain activity in a recognition memory task.[10] The subjects' task was to identify within a list of visually presented words those that were shown for the first time and those that were being repeated. Consistent with other benzodiazepines, oxazepam inhibited the recognition of both new and old words. In contrast kava showed a slightly increased recognition rate and a larger brain response between old and new words. The results of this study once again demonstrate the uncharacteristic effects of kava. In this case, it improves anxiety, but unlike standard anxiety-relieving agents, kava actually improves mental function and, at the recommended levels, does not promote sedation.

How Does Kava Work?

Studies in the 1950s and 1960s showed that the kavalactones exhibit sedative, analgesic, anticonvulsant, and muscle-relaxant effects in laboratory animals. More recent studies have confirmed and/or elaborated on these effects. However, exactly how kava produces these effects is largely unknown. Kava exerts many of its effects by nontraditional mechanisms. For example, most sedative drugs, including the benzodiazepines (e.g., Valium, Halcion, Tranxene, etc.), work by binding to specific receptors (benzodiazepines or GABA receptors) in the brain, which then leads to the neurochemical changes (potentiation of GABA effects), which promote sedation. Studies in animals have shown that the kavalactones do not bind to benzodiazepine or GABA receptors.[4] Instead, the kavalactones are thought to somehow modify the area near the receptor site in a way that enhances GABA binding. However, there are other explanations. For example, studies have indicated that the kavalactones appear to act primarily on the limbic system—the primitive part of the brain that effects all other brain activities and is the principal seat of the emotions and of instinct.[11] It is thought that kava may promote its anxiety-relieving and mood-elevating effects by altering the way in which the limbic system influences emotional processes. Kava is truly a unique antianxiety agent.[12]

An interesting effect of kava compared with many anxiolytic drugs is that unlike the drugs, kava does not lose effectiveness with time. Loss of effectiveness of a drug is known as tolerance. Kavalactones, even when administered in huge amounts in animal studies, demonstrated absolutely no loss of effectiveness.[13]

Dosage

The dosage of kava preparations is based on the level of kavalactones. Based on clinical studies using pure kavalactones or kava extracts standardized for kavalactones, the dosage recommendation for anxiolytic effects is 45 to 70 mg of kavalactones three times daily. For sedative effects, a dosage providing 180 to 210 mg of kavalactones can be taken as a single dose one hour before retiring.

To put the therapeutic dosage in perspective, it is important to point out that a standard bowl of traditionally prepared kava drink contains approximately 250 mg of kavalactones and that several bowls may be consumed at one sitting.

Safety Issues

Although no side effects have been reported using standardized kava extracts at recommended levels in the clinical studies, several case reports have been presented indicating that kava may interfere with dopamine and worsen Parkinson's disease, a condition of decreased dopamine activity in the brain characterized by impaired motor (muscle) function and involuntary muscle twitches.[14] Until this issue is cleared up, kava should not be used in Parkinson's patients.

At a very high dosage (e.g., ten times the dosage recommended), it is possible that kava extracts may produce the same side effects of high kava beverage consumption. High dosages of kava beverage consumed daily over a prolonged period (a few months to a year or more) are associated with "kava dermopathy"—a condition of the skin characterized by a peculiar generalized scaly eruption known as kani.[15] The skin becomes dry and covered with scales, especially the palms of the hand, soles of the feet, forearms, the back, and the shins. It was thought at one time that kava dermopathy may be due to interference with niacin. However, in a double-blind placebo-controlled study no therapeutic effect with niacinamide (100 mg daily) could be demonstrated.[16] It appears the only effective treatment for kava dermopathy is reduction or cessation of kava consumption. Again, no reported cases of kava dermopathy have been noted in individuals taking standardized kava extracts at recommended levels.

Other adverse effects of extremely high doses of kava (e.g., greater than 310 grams per week) for prolonged periods include biochemical abnormalities (low levels of serum albumin, protein, urea, and bilirubin), presence of blood in the urine, increased red blood cell volume, decreased platelet and lymphocyte counts, and shortness of breath.[17] The presence of these adverse effects is questionable because the subjects also reported heavy alcohol and cigarette usage. Nonetheless, high doses of kava are unnecessary and should not be encouraged.

Final Comments

Kava may one day replace benzodiazepines in the pharmacological treatment of anxiety. Kava is able to produce anxiety-relieving effects comparable to benzodiazepines, but is free of the common and expected side effects of these highly addictive drugs. If an individual's depression is associated with a great deal of anxiety, kava extract at the recommended levels can be extremely effective in relieving symptoms.

Chapter 8

Ginkgo Biloba Extract

The extract of Ginkgo biloba leaves standardized to contain 24% ginkgo flavonglycosides and 6% terpenoids may be the most important herbal medicine in the world. It is among the most widely prescribed medicines in both Germany and France, accounting for 1.0% and 1.5%, respectively, of total prescription sales. In 1989 over 100,000 physicians worldwide wrote over 10 million prescriptions for Ginkgo biloba extract. This number is rising rapidly as more physicians and consumers in the United States learn about this important plant medicine. In addition to depression, Ginkgo biloba extract has been shown to be effective in treating the following:

Cerebrovascular insufficiency (insufficient blood flow to
the brain)

Senility (including Alzheimer's disease)

Impotence

Inner ear dysfunction (vertigo, tinnitus, etc.)

Peripheral vascular insufficiency (intermittent claudica-
tion, Raynaud's syndrome, etc.)

Premenstrual syndrome

Retinopathy (macular degeneration, diabetic retinopathy, etc.)

Vascular fragility

Ginkgo's Doctrine of Signature

Throughout history it has been commonly believed that
plants have been signed by the "creator" in some manner to
indicate their therapeutic use. This concept is referred to as
the Doctrine of Signatures. Common examples of this doctrine are: ginseng (*Panax ginseng*), whose root bears strong
resemblance to a human figure and whose general use is as a
tonic; blue cohosh (*Caulophyllum thalictroides*), whose
branches are arranged like limbs in spasm, indicating its use-
fulness in the treatment of muscular spasm; and goldenseal
(*Hydrastis canadensis*), whose yellow-green root signifies its use
in combating jaundice as well as infectious processes. All of
these uses have been confirmed by recent research.

It appears that the Doctrine of Signatures for ginkgo is
its long life and tremendous adaptability to the environment,

indicating that it may promote longevity. The ginkgo is a deciduous tree that is the world's oldest living tree species. The ginkgo tree can be traced back more than 200 million years to the fossils of the Permian period and for this reason is often referred to as "the living fossil."

Once common in North America and Europe, the ginkgo was almost destroyed during the Ice Age in all regions of the world except China, where it has long been cultivated as a sacred tree. The ginkgo tree was brought to America in 1784 to the garden of William Hamilton near Philadelphia. The ginkgo is now planted throughout much of the United States as an ornamental tree. Because ginkgo is the tree most resistant to insects, diseases, and pollution, you will often see it planted along streets in cities.[1]

Ginkgo Extract and Symptoms of Aging

Ginkgo biloba extract has demonstrated remarkably beneficial effects in improving many symptoms associated with aging. Interestingly, the total extract is more active than single isolated components. This suggests synergism between the various components of Ginkgo biloba extract—an explanation that is well supported in more than four hundred clinical and experimental studies utilizing the extract.[1]

Ginkgo biloba extract's primary medical use has been in the treatment of decreased blood flow to the brain and extremities. In over fifty double-blind clinical trials both patients with chronic insufficiency of blood and oxygen to the brain and patients with reduced blood flow to the extremities have responded favorably to Ginkgo biloba extract. The studies have demonstrated Ginkgo biloba extract exerts an extraordinary array of beneficial effects.

Symptoms of decreased blood supply to the brain (cerebrovascular insufficiency) include short-term memory loss, impaired mental performance, dizziness, headache, ringing in the ears, lack of vigilance and depression.[1]

Over forty double-blind controlled studies with Ginkgo biloba extract have shown it to be extremely effective in improving the symptoms of cerebrovascular insufficiency.[2] The quality of research demonstrating this effectiveness is comparable to the quality of research on Hydergine, an FDA-approved drug used in the treatment of cerebrovascular insufficiency and Alzheimer's disease. Eight studies stand out as extremely well designed.[3]

Because Ginkgo biloba extract increases brain blood flow and oxygen supply to the brain, it offers significant protection against strokes and aids in recovery from a stroke.[4]

Ginkgo biloba extract also increases the rate at which information is transmitted at the nerve cell level.[5] Since memory is dependent upon the transmission of the nerve signal, this mechanism may play a key role in the memory-enhancing effects of Ginkgo biloba extract.[6]

Table 8.1 Characteristics of Well-Conducted Controlled Trials

Trial	Indication Duration of symptoms Average age	Daily dose/ Duration of treatment
Schmidt, 1991	Cerebral insufficiency 26 months 59 years	150 mg/12 weeks
Bruchert, 1991	Cerebral insufficiency 46 months 69 years	150 mg/12 weeks
Meyer, 1986	Tinnitus, dizziness, hearing impairment 4–5 months 50 years	16 mg (4 ml)/3 months
Taillandier, 1986	Cerebral insufficiency 5 years 82 years	160 mg/12 months
Haguenauer, 1986	Vertiginous syndrome and tinnitus, headaches, nausea, hearing loss 21 weeks 50 years	160 mg/3 months
Vorberg, 1989	Cerebral insufficiency 21 months 70 years	112 mg/12 weeks
Eckmann, 1990	Cerebral insufficiency 32 months 55 years	160 mg/6 weeks
Wesnes, 1987	Mild idiopathic cognitive impairment 71 years	120 mg/12 weeks

1. No.* randomized 2. No. analyzed	Endpoints	Results
1. 50/49 2. 50/49	1. 12 symptoms; OS(4) 2. Overall assessment doctor; OS(3) 3. Overall assessment patient; OS(3)	1. Significant differences for 8 of 12 2. 72% vs 8% improved 3. 70% vs 14% improved
1. 156/157 2. 110/99	1. 12 symptoms; OS(4) 2. Overall assessment doctor; OS(3) 3. Overall assessment patient; OS(3)	1. Significant differences for 8 of 12 2. 71% vs 32% improved 3. 83% vs 53% improved
1. 58/45 (?) 2. 55/45 (?)	1. Symptoms; OS(4) 2. Overall assessment; days to improvement or cure	1. Significant difference for intensity; positive trend for discomfort 2. 70 days vs. 119 days
1. 101/109 2. 80/86	1. Scale for geriatric patients (17 items); change from randomization after 3 months 2. After 6 months 3. After 9 months 4. After 12 months	1. 10% vs. 4% 2. 15% vs. 4% 3. 15% vs. 8% 4. 17% vs. 8%
1. 35/35 2. 34/33	1. Symptoms; VAS and others 2. Overall assessment doctor; OS(5)	1. Vertigo: 75% vs. 18% beneficial change 2. 47% vs. 18% symptoms disappeared
1. 50/50 2. 49/47	6 symptoms; OS(4)	1. Concentration: 54% vs. 19% improved 2. Memory: 52% vs. 17% improved 3. Anxiety: 48% vs. 17% improved 4. Dizziness: 61% vs. 23% improved 5. Headache: 65% vs. 24% improved 6. Tinnitus: 37% vs. 12% improved
1. 30/30 2. 29/29	12 symptoms; OS(4)	Significant differences for 11 of 12 symptoms after 4 and 6 weeks
1. 28/30 2. 27/27	1. Cognitive test battery 2. Behavioral rating scale 3. VAS mood 4. Overall assessment doctor and patient	1. Significant differences for combined scores 2. No differences 3. No significant differences 4. No differences, nearly all patients improved

*Ginkgo/placebo   OS(4) = 4-point ordinal scale; VAS = visual analog scale

A Case History with Ginkgo

Helen presented complaints common to most people seventy-four years of age: dizziness, ringing in the ear, poor short-term memory, and a general lack of enthusiasm for life. Most elderly people accept these symptoms as simply a sign of old age. What brought Helen in to see me was more than just these symptoms. When I first saw her in October 1992, she had just had a small stroke the month before. Fortunately there was no permanent damage. The stroke scared her. It would scare anyone. Her M.D. placed her immediately on a drug called coumadin. This drug prevents her platelets from clumping together to form a blood clot by interfering with the body's ability to utilize vitamin K.

She was having trouble with the drug. Common side effects such as easy bruising and the breaking of blood capillaries are thought of as minor inconveniences necessary to endure in order to obtain the benefits of the drug. However, Helen was experiencing a real sensitivity to the drug and was bleeding from the nose and gastrointestinal tract. She had to be taken off the drug. Usually a medical alternative for many people in Helen's situation is aspirin. But Helen had a history of stomach ulcers and was extremely sensitive to aspirin's tendency to cause ulcers.

She was in a difficult situation. She was recovering from a stroke, yet was likely to experience another one if she did not take steps to improve the blood supply to the brain as well as inhibit the formation of blood clots. Fortunately, one of her friends was a patient of mine. She told Helen all about the benefits she had experienced from Ginkgo biloba extract and shared with Helen an article I had written for a health magazine.

Intrigued but not yet convinced, Helen made an appointment to see me. I explained to her that strokes are most often due to a buildup of cholesterol within the arteries supplying blood to the brain—the carotid arteries. A clot can form if the blood supply is slowed by the buildup of plaque. Although the blood clot may be new, the process that promoted the clot formation is basically the end-stage of long-term problem—atherosclerosis. Many people either die from a stroke or suffer permanent handicaps. Helen was in the lucky group who survive a stroke with no lasting ill effects. She had an opportunity to use the experience in a positive way by adopting a diet, lifestyle, and natural program designed to add not only years to her life but life to her years.

If patients are at extremely high risk of having another stroke, I think the standard recommendation of coumadin and aspirin is a good idea. However, while focusing on preventing blood clots, this therapy does not provide the myriad of benefits that Ginkgo biloba extract does. Ginkgo biloba extract not only inhibits platelets from forming blood clots, it enhances blood and oxygen supply to the brain—a critical goal in helping aid recovery from a stroke. Since Helen was still demonstrating symptoms of cerebrovascular insufficiency, Ginkgo appeared to be a perfect recommendation. However, it was not the only recommendation I gave. I also recommended my standard nutritional supplementation program of a high-potency multiple vitamin and mineral formula (Doctor's Choice for Women from Enzymatic Therapy), extra antioxidants (Doctor's Choice Antioxidant Formula from Enzymatic Therapy), and one tablespoon of Barlean's High Lignan Flax Oil.

It is often difficult to describe in words the changes I see in people. When I first saw Helen, she looked old. I would say she looked like a dim light bulb. One month later, however, she looked vibrant and radiant. She reported that she felt better than she had in years, her dizziness was gone, and she seemed to be functioning better mentally. She was exuberant and very happy. Helen's response is typical of most elderly people's response to Ginkgo biloba extract. Typically, one of the major changes that Ginkgo tends to promote is an improved outlook on life.

Ginkgo Biloba Extract Relieves Depression in the Elderly

Researchers began studying the antidepressive effects of Ginkgo biloba extract as a result of the improvement in mood noted by patients suffering from cerebrovascular insufficiency in double-blind studies. In one of the more recent double-blind studies, forty elderly patients with depression (ranging from fifty-one to seventy-eight years of age) who had not benefited fully from standard antidepressant drugs were given either 80 mg of Ginkgo biloba extract three times daily or a placebo.[7] By the end of the four-week study, the total score of the Hamilton Depression Scale was reduced from an average of 14 to 7. At the end of the eight-week study, the total score in the Ginkgo biloba extract group had dropped to 4.5. By comparison, the placebo group dropped from 14 to only 13. This study indicates that Ginkgo biloba extract can be used with standard antidepressants and it may enhance their effectiveness, particularly in patients over fifty years of age.

In addition to human studies, Ginkgo biloba extract has also demonstrated antidepressant effects in a number of animal models including the learned-helplessness model. The most interesting of these studies demonstrated that Ginkgo biloba extract was able to counteract one of the major changes in brain chemistry associated with aging—the reduction in the number of serotonin receptor sites.[8] Typically, as people age there is a significant reduction in the number of serotonin receptor sites on brain cells. As a result, the elderly are more susceptible to depression, impaired mental function, insomnia, and sleep disturbances. The study was designed to determine whether Ginkgo biloba extract could alter the number of serotonin receptors in aged (twenty-four-month-old) and young (four-month-old) rats. At the beginning of the study the older rats had a 22 percent lower number of serotonin binding sites compared with the younger rats. The results of chronic treatment with Ginkgo biloba extract for twenty-one consecutive days demonstrated that there was no change in receptor binding in young rats, but in the aged rats there was a statistically significant increase (by 33 percent) in the number of serotonin-binding sites. These results indicate that

Ginkgo biloba extract may counteract at least some, if not all, of the age–dependent reductions of serotonin binding sites in the aging human brain as well.

The exact mechanism to explain Ginkgo biloba extract's effect on increasing serotonin receptors has not yet been determined; however, Ginkgo biloba extract may address two major reasons why serotonin receptors decline with aging: (a) impaired receptor synthesis; or (b) changes in cerebral neuronal membranes or receptors as a result of free radical damage. Ginkgo biloba extract has demonstrated an ability to increase protein synthesis. In addition, Ginkgo biloba extract is known to be a potent antioxidant. The most likely explanation is that it is the combination of these two effects (and others) rather than one single mechanism.

Dosage

Most of the clinical research on Ginkgo biloba has utilized a standardized extract, containing 24% Ginkgo flavonglycosides (heterosides), at a dose of 40 mg three times a day. However, some studies have used a higher dosage of 80 mg three times daily.

It is difficult to devise a dosage schedule using other forms of Ginkgo due to extreme variation in the content of active compounds in dried leaf and crude extracts. Whatever form of Ginkgo is used, it appears to be essential that it be standardized for content and activity. For example, a standard 1:5 tincture obtained from the highest possible flavonoid-content crude ginkgo leaf would require 1 ounce of the tincture per day to provide the equivalent dosage level of the standardized extract.

Clinical research clearly shows that Ginkgo biloba extract should be taken consistently for at least twelve weeks in order to determine effectiveness. Although most people report benefits within two to three weeks, some may take longer to respond.

Safety Issues

Ginkgo biloba extract is extremely safe, and side effects are uncommon. In forty-four double-blind studies involving 9,772 patients taking Ginkgo biloba extract, the number of side effects reported was extremely small. The most common side effect, gastrointestinal discomfort, occurred in only twenty-one cases, followed by headache (seven cases) and dizziness (six cases).[1]

In contrast to the tolerance of the leaf extract, contact with or ingestion of the fruit pulp has produced severe allergic reactions.[9] Contact with the fruit pulp causes erythema and edema, with the rapid formation of vesicles accompanied by severe itching. This is similar to an allergic reaction to the poison ivy–oak–sumac group, suggesting cross-reactivity between Ginkgo biloba fruit and this family. Ingestion of as little as two pieces of fruit pulp has been reported to cause severe gastrointestinal irritation from the mouth to the anus.

Final Comments

I recommend Ginkgo biloba extract to all my patients over the age of fifty. There are several reasons for this recommendation. In addition to the possibility that Ginkgo biloba extract may prevent the age-related decline in serotonin receptors, the main reason is that Ginkgo biloba extract appears to offer some protection against Alzheimer's disease. Have you ever had someone close to you develop Alzheimer's disease? If you have, you know firsthand about this devastating experience. In experimental studies in animal models of Alzheimer's disease, Ginkgo biloba extract has shown impressive results in preventing the disease. Although it remains to be proven that Ginkgo biloba extract offers the same degree of prevention in humans, given the excellent safety profile of Ginkgo biloba extract along with the glimmer of hope, it certainly seems like a good idea to take 40 mg of Ginkgo biloba extract three times daily as a preventive measure.

Preliminary studies in established Alzheimer's patients are quite promising. Ginkgo biloba extract can help delay and in some cases reverse the mental deterioration in the early stages of Alzheimer's disease. Results from a recent double-blind study offer additional support.[10] Ginkgo biloba extract may help to enable the patient to maintain a normal life for a while and avoid being put in a nursing home.

In the study, forty patients with a preliminary diagnosis

of senile dementia of the Alzheimer's type received either 80 mg of Ginkgo biloba extract or placebo three times daily for three months. Patients were assessed by standard tests including the SKT, Sandoz Clinical Assessment Geriatric Scale, and EEG at baseline and at one, two, and three months. Results indicated that Ginkgo biloba extract improved all parameters, usually in the first month, compared with the placebo. Consistent with other studies with Ginkgo biloba extract, the longer Ginkgo biloba extract is used, the more obvious the benefits become. Ginkgo biloba extract was well tolerated and no side effects were noted in the trial.

Another natural compound showing promise in depression in the elderly, impaired mental function, and Alzheimer's disease is phosphatidylserine—the major phospholipid (see page 126) in the brain.[11] The fluidity of brain cell membranes is dependent upon adequate phosphatidylserine. Normally the brain can manufacture sufficient levels of phosphatidylserine, but if there is a deficiency of SAM (discussed in Chapter 9) or essential fatty acids, the brain may not be able to make sufficient phosphatidylserine. Since SAM levels and folic acid are inadequate in depression, it is likely that insufficient phosphatidylserine synthesis will occur.

Phosphatidylserine supplementation can produce very good results in improving mental function and depression in the elderly.[11] In the largest double-blind study with phosphatidylserine, a total of 494 elderly patients (aged between sixty-five and ninety-three years) with moderate to severe senility were given either phosphatidylserine or a placebo for six months.[12] The patients were assessed for mental performance, behavior, and mood at the beginning and end of the study. Statistically significant improvements were noted in the phosphatidylserine-treated group in mental function, mood, and behavior.

In a double-blind study of depressed elderly patients, phosphatidylserine was shown to improve depressive symptoms, memory, and behavior.[13] Phosphatidylserine promoted this improvement without influencing monoamine metabolism, suggesting another mechanism of action. Improved brain cell membrane fluidity may be one explanation. Another is the fact that phosphatidylserine has been shown to reduce cortisol secretion in response to stress.[14]

Even though phosphatidylserine appears to be of great value to elderly patients, I do not recommend it that often. The reason? The price. A month's dose of 100 mg three times per day costs about $75 per month. I am hoping this price comes down. In the meantime what I have my patients do instead is take Ginkgo biloba extract as well as provide the necessary nutrients their brain will need to manufacture phosphatidylserine—essential fatty acid (particularly the omega-3 oils), folic acid, vitamin B12, and vitamin C.

Chapter 9

Amino Acids

Several amino acids, the individual building-block units of protein, function as neurotransmitters or precursors to neurotransmitters. The use of monoamine precursors, particularly tryptophan and tyrosine, has offered a more "natural way" of influencing monoamine metabolism compared to antidepressant drugs. Amino-acid therapy has been shown to be as effective as antidepressant drugs. This chapter will review the data on tryptophan, tyrosine and phenylalanine, S-adenosyl-methionine, and GABA.

Tryptophan

For more than thirty years, L-tryptophan was used by thousands of people in the United States and around the world safely and effectively for insomnia and depression. But in October 1989, some people taking tryptophan started reporting strange symptoms to physicians—severe muscle and joint pain, high fever, weakness, swelling of the arms and legs, and shortness of breath. The syndrome was dubbed EMS (eosinophilia-myalgia syndrome). Virtually all cases of tryptophan-induced EMS could be traced to one manufacturer, Showa Denko. Of the six Japanese companies that supplied tryptophan to the United States, Showa Denko was the largest in that it supplied 50 to 60 percent of all the tryptophan being used in the United States. Due to a change in manufacturing procedures, Showa Denko's tryptophan produced from October 1988 to June 1989 became contaminated with a substance now linked to EMS.[1]

Tryptophan has remained off the market despite the fact that, before the Showa Denko incident, it had been used safely for decades. There are numerous examples of contaminated foods and medicines causing health problems and even death. Yet in most industries, once the problem of contamination is solved, manufacturers are once again allowed to market their products whether it is contaminated grapes, bottled water, or hamburgers. But for some reason tryptophan has not been allowed back in health food stores even though the contamination issue is resolved.

The information presented below on tryptophan is presented with the hope that the FDA will allow uncontaminated tryptophan to once again be sold in health food stores.

Tryptophan is the precursor to serotonin and melatonin (discussed in the next chapter). The level of serotonin and melatonin in the brain is dependent on how much tryptophan is in the blood and how much of that tryptophan is transported from the blood into the brain across the blood–brain barrier.[2] Since tryptophan levels in the blood are typically reduced, it is safe to assume that tryptophan, serotonin, and melatonin levels in the brain are also lower. The basic theory of tryptophan supplementation in depression (and insomnia) is that it will increase the level of serotonin and melatonin in the brain. Although most researchers have concerned themselves with serotonin, melatonin is also a significant factor.

In addition to low tryptophan levels in the blood, there is evidence that tryptophan transport across the blood–brain barrier may also be inhibited in depressed patients. A tryptophan metabolite (kynurenine), several other amino acids, and insulin insensitivity all inhibit transport of tryptophan into the brain. Tryptophan shares the transport system with leucine, isoleucine, valine, tyrosine, and phenylalanine. The quantity of these other amino acids in food is usually much greater than the amount of tryptophan. Therefore a protein-rich meal will result in decreased brain tryptophan uptake. By contrast, a carbohydrate meal will result in increased tryptophan uptake into the brain because of the lack of competing amino acids and the effects of insulin.[2]

Supplementation with L-tryptophan in depressed patients has resulted in mixed results.[3] There are many factors to consider when looking at these studies, such as study size, duration, and dosage. Regarding dosage, it is important to realize that a number of factors, such as estrogens and corticosteroids, as well as tryptophan, stimulate the activity of tryptophan oxygenase. When activated, this enzyme results in less tryptophan being delivered to the brain. Tryptophan at dosages greater than 6 grams a day could actually lead to decreased brain tryptophan levels.

Vitamin B_6 supplementation (50 mg to 100 mg daily) can decrease this effect by decreasing kynurenine levels.[2] Another vitamin that can help increase brain tryptophan levels is niacinamide (vitamin B_3). Niacinamide has been used in conjunction with tryptophan in several clinical studies. It appears that the use of tryptophan alone as the sole therapy is not as effective as when used in conjunction with other critical nutrients, and in some cases may not be effective when used alone.

Phenylalanine and Tyrosine

Although the number of clinical studies that utilized phenylalanine or tyrosine for depression does not approach the number that used tryptophan, there is evidence that these monoamine precursors may be effective in some individuals.[4]

Phenylalanine, besides being converted to tyrosine, can be converted to phenylethylamine (PEA). This compound has amphetaminelike stimulant properties and is suggested to be an endogenous stimulatory or antidepressive substance in humans. (Note: This biogenic amine is found in high concentrations in chocolate, which might explain the latter's addictiveness.)

Low urinary PEA levels are found in depressed patients, while high levels are found in schizophrenia. Phenylalanine, both D and L-forms, has been demonstrated to increase urinary PEA output and central-nervous-system PEA concentrations. As phenylalanine inhibits the conversion of tyrosine to L-DOPA (it inhibits the enzyme tyrosine hydroxylase), supplementation with phenylalanine will result in higher PEA levels.

Conversely, the antidepressant activity of supplemental tyrosine may also be related to its increasing PEA, octopamine, and tyramine. The fact that tyrosine is converted to L-DOPA and studies in depressed patients taking L-DOPA alone have not shown any benefit tends to substantiate this assumption.

Like tryptophan, the brain tyrosine and phenylalanine content is best determined by the ratio of serum tyrosine concentration to the sum of its brain-uptake competitors, that is, leucine, isoleucine, valine, and tryptophan.[4] Unlike tryptophan, tyrosine ratios are increased by high-protein meals.

Table 9.1 summarizes clinical studies using phenylalanine

Table 9.1 Phenylalanine and Tyrosine in Depression

Reference	Number Patients	Dose (mg/day)	Duration (days)	Clinical Effects and Comments
Yaryura et al. [1974]	15	200–400	14	(d,l–P) 10 severely depressed patients responded
Fischer et al. [1975]	23	100	1–13	(d, or d,l–P) A complete response was observed in 17 patients previously unresponsive to tricyclics and MAO inhibitors
Beckman et al. [1977]	20	75–200	20	(d,l–P) 8 complete remissions, 4 marked improvement; used Hamilton Depression Scale and von Zerssen Self-rating Questionnaire
Heller [1978]	55	100–400	60–180	(d–P) 73% recovered completely after 15 days, 23% had marked improvement, 4% failed to respond

Heller [1978]	60	100	30	(d–P) Complete remission and improvement 83% for the phenylalanine group compared to 73% for the imipramine group; double-blind controlled study—no diagnostic criteria or rating scales were reported
Beckman [1979]	27	200	30	(d,l–P) No significant difference between phenylalanine and imipramine groups
Gibson et al. [1983]	9	300	ongoing	(T) Double-blind, placebo-controlled study; tyrosine demonstrated a rate of response (60–70%) typical of most major antidepressants without side effects

From: Beckman, H.: Phenylalanine in affective disorders. *Adv. Biol. Psychiatry* 10:137–47, 1983. And: Gibson, C., and Gelenberg, A.: Tyrosine for depression. *Adv. Biol. Psychiatry* 10:148–59, 1983.

P = Phenylalanine, T = Tyrosine

and/or tyrosine for depression. These results indicate that phenylalanine and tyrosine supplementation produce results comparable to antidepressant drugs without the side effects.

S-Adenosyl-Methionine (SAM)

SAM was discussed briefly in Chapter 5. It functions closely with folic acid and vitamin B_{12} in "methylation" reactions. Methylation is the process of adding a single carbon unit (a methyl group) to another molecule. SAM is many times more effective in transferring methyl groups than folic acid. SAM is involved in the methylation of monoamines, neurotransmitters, and phospholipids such as phosphatidylcholine and phosphatidylserine. As discussed on page 165, phosphatidylserine has demonstrated significant antidepressive effects in the elderly and has shown an ability to improve mental function in the early stages of Alzheimer's disease.

Normally the brain manufactures all the SAM it needs from the amino acid methionine. However, SAM synthesis is impaired in depressed patients. Supplementing the diet with SAM in depressed patients results in increased levels of serotonin, dopamine, and phosphatides, and improved binding of neurotransmitters to receptor sites, resulting in increased serotonin and dopamine activity and improved brain cell membrane fluidity resulting in significant clinical improvement.[5]

The antidepressive effects of folic acid discussed on page 118 are mild compared with the effects noted in clinical trials using SAM. Unfortunately, as of this writing (October 1995), SAM is still not available in the United States. I am including this description of SAM because I believe it will be introduced into U.S. health food stores as a nutritional supplement in the very near future. Based on results from a number of clinical studies, it appears that SAM is perhaps the most effective natural antidepressant.[6] Tables 9.2 and 9.3 summarize double-blind studies comparing SAM with either a placebo or a tricyclic drug such as imipramine.

The studies cited in Tables 9.2 and 9.3 utilized injectable SAM. However, more recent studies using a new oral preparation at a dosage of 400 mg four times daily (1600 mg total) have demonstrated that SAM is just as effective orally as it is when given intravenously.[7] SAM is better tolerated and has a quicker onset of antidepressant action compared with tricyclic antidepressants.

The most recent study compared SAM with the tricyclic desipramine. In addition to clinical response, the blood level of SAM was determined in both groups. At the end of the four-week trial, 62 percent of the patients treated with SAM and 50 percent of the patients treated with desipramine had significantly improved. Regardless of the type of treatment, patients with a 50 percent decrease in their Hamilton Depression Scale (HAMD) score showed a significant increase in plasma SAM concentration. These results suggest that one of the ways that tricyclic drugs exert antidepressive effects is by raising SAM levels.[8]

No significant side effects have been reported with oral SAM. However, because SAM can cause nausea and vomit-

Table 9.2   Double-Blind Clinical Studies with SAM Versus Placebo in Depression

Authors	SAM Responders	Placebo Responders	Conclusion
Fazio et al. [1973]	Not quantified		SAM superior to placebo based on Hamilton Depression Scale
Agnoli et al. [1976]	20/20	1/10	SAM superior to placebo (100% response in SAM group, 10% in placebo)
Muscettola et al. [1982]	4/10	0/10	SAM superior to placebo
Janicak [1982]	5/7	0/5	SAM superior to placebo
Caruso et al. [1984]	Not quantified		SAM superior to placebo based on Hamilton Depression Scale
Carney et al. [1986]	Not quantified		SAM superior to placebo based on Hamilton Depression Scale & Beck Scale
De Leo [1987]	Not quantified		SAM superior to placebo based on Clinical Global Impression Scale
Total	29/37 (78%)	1/25 (4%)	SAM dramatically more effective than placebo

ing in some people, it is recommended that SAM be started at a dosage of 200 mg twice daily for the first day, increased to 400 mg twice daily on day three, then 400 mg three times daily on day ten, and finally to the full dosage of 400 mg four times daily after twenty days.

Individuals with bipolar (manic) depression should not take SAM. Because of SAM antidepressant activity individuals with bipolar depression are susceptible to experiencing hypomania or mania (see page 17 for definitions). This effect is exclusive to some individuals with bipolar depression.

GABA

Benzodiazepine drugs such as Valium work by stimulating receptors in the brain for gamma-aminobutyric acid (GABA)—the brain's natural calming agent. Although GABA is manufactured from the amino acid glutamine in the brain, in some cases of anxiety, panic disorders, and depression the brain does not make enough GABA.

Although to my knowledge there are no clinical trials of GABA in anxiety, GABA has been used with reported success at the famed Princeton Brain Bio Center. Eric Braverman, M.D., and Carl Pfeiffer, M.D., reported in their book *The Healing Nutrients Within: Facts, Findings and New Research on Amino Acids* that GABA has been used in a variety of brain disorders including epilepsy and schizophrenia. For anxiety, these experts recommend that GABA be used in severely anx-

Table 9.3   Double-Blind Clinical Studies with SAM Versus Antidepressant Drugs in Depression

Authors	SAM Responders	Drug Responders	Conclusion
Mantero et al. [1975]	11/16	9/15	SAM comparable to imipramine (75 mg/day)
Barberi et al. [1978]	10/10	8/10	SAM more effective than amitriptyline (100 mg/day)
Del Vecchio et al. [1978]	5/14	4/10	SAM comparable to clomipramine (100 mg/day)
Miccoli et al. [1978]	35/45	30/41	SAM comparable to clomipramine (100 mg/day)
Scarzella et al. [1978]	9/10	9/10	SAM comparable to clomipramine (100 mg/day)
Scaggion et al. [1982]	18/22	10/18	SAM more effective to nomifensine (200 mg/day)
Kufferle et al. [1982]	7/9	6/9	SAM comparable to clomipramine (50 mg/day)

Plotkin [1988]	9/9	2/9	SAM more effective than imipramine (150 mg/day)
Janicak [1988]	5/7	2/3	SAM comparable to imipramine (150 mg/day)
Total	109/142	80/124	SAM is significantly more effective than antidepressant drugs.
	76%	61%	

From: Janicak, P.G., et al.: Parenteral S-adenosylmethionine in depression. A literature review and preliminary report. *Psychopharmacol. Bull.* 25:238–41, 1989.

ious individuals addicted to benzodiazepines at a dosage of 200 mg four times daily.[9]

Final Comments

Amino acid therapy can produce dramatic results in depressed individuals. A great deal of clinical research documents the effectiveness of tryptophan and SAM. Unfortunately tryptophan is not currently available because of a past contamination problem, and SAM is not yet available due primarily to price considerations (i.e., SAM is available as a raw material, but it is very expensive). Hopefully, these natural medicines will be available to be used with confidence in the very near future.

Phenylalanine, tyrosine, and GABA are available commercially. Recommendations for their use are given in the next chapter.

Chapter 10

Melatonin

Melatonin became an overnight sensation after it was featured as the cover story in the August 7, 1995, *Newsweek*. The article discussed the potential of melatonin in relieving insomnia, jet lag, stress, and depression as well as fighting cancer, boosting the immune system, preventing heart disease, and acting as an antioxidant. The *Newsweek* article precipitated a mad rush to health food stores to buy this "wonder pill." However, some caution is warranted. This chapter shall discuss the benefits and possible detriments of melatonin.

What Is Melatonin?

Melatonin (not to be confused with melanin, the compound responsible for skin pigment) is a hormone manufactured from serotonin and secreted by the pineal gland. The pineal gland, a small pea-sized gland at the base of the brain, has been a source of curiosity since antiquity. The ancient Greeks considered the pineal gland the seat of the soul, a concept that was extended by the philosopher Descartes. In the seventeenth and eighteenth centuries physicians associated "madness" with the pineal gland. Physicians in the early 1900s believed the pineal gland was somehow involved with the endocrine system. The identification of melatonin in 1958 provided the first solid scientific evidence of an essential role of the pineal gland. It is now thought that the sole function of the pineal gland is to manufacture and secrete melatonin.

The exact function of melatonin is still poorly understood, but it is critically involved in the synchronization of hormone secretion. The natural biorhythm of hormone secretion is referred to as the circadian rhythm. The human body is governed by an internal clock that signals the secretion of various hormones at different times to regulate body functions. Melatonin plays a key role as the biological time keeper of hormone secretion. Melatonin also helps control periods of sleepiness and wakefulness. Release of melatonin is stimulated by darkness and is suppressed by light.

In the discussion of the treatment of seasonal affective disorder with light therapy on pages 18–19, it was mentioned that the antidepressant effect of light therapy is probably due to balancing of the altered circadian rhythm by restoring proper melatonin synthesis and secretion by the pineal gland. Disruption of pineal function is thought to be a major reason for seasonal affective disorder as well as jet lag.[1]

Several double-blind studies have shown melatonin to be very effective in relieving jet lag.[2] Different dosage recommendations have been given. Some researchers have recommended that melatonin be taken at the beginning of the sleep period at the point of departure starting a few days before departure (especially when traveling eastward). Others have recommended taking melatonin just one time on the first evening upon arriving at the new destination. The latter recommendation avoids the problem of extreme drowsiness sometimes produced by melatonin at an unwanted time; for example, if I were planning to fly to Rome, I would take the melatonin at one P.M. for three days prior to my trip.

A recent study was designed to answer the question of optimal timing of melatonin supplementation.[3] In the study, fifty-two members of an airline cabin crew flying an international route were randomly assigned to three groups; early melatonin (5 mg started three days prior to arrival until five days after return home); late melatonin (placebo for three days then 5 mg melatonin for five days at new destination); and placebo. Daily ratings in jet lag, mood, and sleepiness measures demonstrated the best recovery was in the late-melatonin group. The early-melatonin group actually demonstrated a worse recovery compared with the placebo group. This study suggests the best way to use melatonin for jet lag is 5 mg in the evening at the new destination for five days.

Melatonin and Depression

Initial studies performed in the 1980s demonstrated that melatonin levels are typically below normal in patients with clinical depression.[4] However, in all of these studies it turned out that antidepressant drugs or other factors were responsible for the depressed melatonin levels. More recent studies have not supported the association of low melatonin levels being common in patients with clinical depression.[5] These studies measured melatonin levels in drug-free, depressed patients and were careful to match these subjects with a control group to compare melatonin levels against. In addition, it has been demonstrated that normal subjects secreting no melatonin do not frequently suffer from depression.[1]

Initially it was thought that melatonin may affect mood as a result of reducing cortisol levels by inhibiting the secretion by the pituitary hormone ACTH, which then signals the adrenal glands to secrete cortisol. With melatonin deficiency, cortisol levels would be expected to be increased. This appears to be the case in many depressed patients, as both decreased melatonin and increased cortisol concentrations are frequently found.[4] However, it is unlikely that melatonin supplementation can significantly reduce cortisol levels, as research has shown melatonin supplementation does not suppress either ACTH or cortisol secretion.[6] What all this data indicates is that melatonin is unlikely to produce any significant positive effects in the treatment of depression in most patients. Clinical research seems to bear this out. In fact, one double-blind study conducted in 1973 demonstrated that melatonin supplementation actually dramatically worsened clinical depression in some cases.[7] Obviously, worsening of depression is quite serious, as it increases the risk for suicide. A possible explanation for the worsening is the fact that the melatonin was given two to four times during the day—a time when melatonin levels are typically low. Another study in nondepressed subjects demonstrated that when melatonin was given during the day, it tended to cause fatigue, confusion, and sleepiness.[8]

Melatonin and Insomnia

Melatonin plays an important role in the induction of sleep. Low melatonin secretion at night can be a cause of insomnia. Several double-blind trials have shown melatonin supplementation to be very effective in promoting sleep.[9] However, some studies showed melatonin had no effect on sleep even if the dosage was very high (e.g., 75 mg or 150 mg).[10] It appears that the sleep-promoting effects of melatonin are only apparent if melatonin levels are low.[11] In other words, melatonin is not like taking a sleeping pill. It will only produce its effects when melatonin levels are low. When melatonin is given just before going to bed in normal subjects or in patients with insomnia who have normal melatonin levels, it produces no sedative effect. That is because normally just prior to going to bed there is a rise in melatonin secretion. Melatonin supplementation is only effective as a sedative when the pineal gland's own production of melatonin is very low. Two groups in whom low melatonin is extremely common are the elderly and the depressed.

Dosage

Melatonin is appropriate for supplementation when low melatonin levels are suspected. The amount of melatonin necessary to produce benefit in these cases is largely unknown. A dosage of 3 mg at bedtime is more than enough, as dosages as low as 0.1 mg and 0.3 mg have been shown to produce a sedative effect when melatonin levels are low.[12] The urinary excretion rate for melatonin is approximately 0.03 mg per twenty-four hours.[13]

Safety Issues

Although there appear to be no serious side effects at recommended dosages, conceivably melatonin supplementation could disrupt the normal circadian rhythm. In one study a daily dosage of 8 mg a day for only four days resulted in significant alteration in circadian rhythm.[6] It is not known what sort of effect would occur at commonly recommended dosages (i.e., 3 mg). In addition, as noted above, in some cases of depression the patients got much worse when they were given melatonin during the day.

Final Comments

In my opinion melatonin is not suitable for indiscriminate use. Melatonin may benefit some patients with depression or insomnia and is suitable for treating jet lag. However, melatonin is an important regulating hormone. The National Nutritional Foods Association (a supplement industry trade group) has advised supplement manufacturers and health food stores that melatonin "may be inappropriate as a product to be sold in a health-food store," and many health food stores have taken it off the shelves. I view these measures as being extremely responsible. While I am a strong advocate of self-care, because of potential complications with inappropriate use I feel that melatonin is best utilized when it is prescribed by a licensed health care practitioner. There is a lot of hype right now about melatonin. Some of it is appropriate, but remember, melatonin is a hormone, not a nutrient.

Chapter 11

Putting It
All Together

If you have made it this far, you may be a little confused as to what exactly you need to do. This chapter will help guide you to the natural alternatives that should provide the greatest benefit to you.

General Guidelines

The following seven recommendations are appropriate for everyone with depression. Adopting these guidelines is all that the majority of people with depression will need to do to elevate their mood.

1. Develop a positive, optimistic mental attitude by
    Setting goals
    Using positive self-talk and affirmations
    Asking yourself empowering questions
    Seeking the help of a mental health professional
2. Rule out an organic or physiological cause of depression, as described in Chapter 3.
3. If you smoke, get help to quit.
4. Avoid the intake of caffeine, other stimulants, and alcohol.
5. Exercise regularly.
6. Perform a relaxation/stress-reduction technique for ten to fifteen minutes each day.
7. Find ways to interject humor and laughter in your life.

ADDITIONAL RECOMMENDATIONS FOR DEPRESSION

If you are currently taking Prozac or another antidepressant, please consult your physician to discuss the appropriateness of using the natural antidepressants discussed in this book. I recommend that these natural antidepressants be used as "crutches" until the dietary, lifestyle, and psychological therapies take hold. Most people will not need this support. If you find that you do, here are my recommendations:

- If you are over 50, take Ginkgo biloba extract at a dosage of 80 mg three times daily. Also, I would recommend taking an additional 1,200 mcg of folic acid and 1,200 mcg of vitamin B_{12} daily.
- If you are under 50, take St. John's wort extract (0.3% hypericin content) at a dosage of 300 mg three times daily.

- If additional support is needed, take 2,000 mg of D- or L-phenylalanine or 1,000 mg of L-tyrosine upon arising in the morning, before breakfast.

FOR ANXIETY

If anxiety is more of a problem than depression, take kava extract at a dosage sufficient to provide 60 mg of kavalactones three times daily, or GABA at a dosage of 200 mg four times daily. (Note: Kava and GABA can be used together.)

FOR INSOMNIA

You may respond to melatonin. Try taking 3 mg before going to bed. If this does not work, follow one of the following recommendations:

- Try taking valerian extract. Valerian (*Valeriana officinalis*) has been widely used in folk medicine as a sedative. Recent scientific studies have substantiated valerian's ability to improve sleep quality and relieve insomnia without side effects.[1] The best results are obtained by using valerian extracts standardized to contain 0.8% valeric acid at a dosage of 150–300 mg thirty minutes before going to bed.
- Take 200 to 400 mg of GABA thirty minutes before going to bed.

Final Comments

If you would like to contact a naturopath (N.D.) or holistic medical doctor (M.D.) or osteopath (D.O.), contact either the American Association of Naturopathic Physicians or the

American Holistic Medical Association. The American Association of Naturopathic Physicians (AANP) is the professional organization of licensed naturopathic physicians. It is seeking to expand licensure of naturopaths in individual states and provinces. Although naturopaths practice in virtually every state and Canadian province, currently only Alaska, Alberta, Arizona, British Columbia, Connecticut, District of Columbia, Hawaii, Manitoba, Montana, Ontario, Oregon, Saskatchewan, and Washington offer licensure to naturopaths. The organization is also seeking to differentiate the professional trained naturopath from the unscrupulous individual claiming to be a naturopath just because he or she received a "mail order" degree. For more information and a referral service, contact:

The American Association of Naturopathic Physicians
P.O. Box 20386
Seattle, WA 98102
(206) 323-7610

The American Holistic Medical Association is composed of medical doctors, osteopaths and naturopaths who share a common philosophy of encouraging personal responsibility for health and emphasizing the whole person.

American Holistic Medical Association
4101 Lake Boone Trail #201
Raleigh, NC 26707
(919) 787-5146

Another organization that may be of help is the Academy for Guided Imagery. This organization certifies health professionals in guided imagery. If you are having trouble learning how to relax or perform visualization exercises, contact the Academy for Guided Imagery for an expert in your area:

The Academy for Guided Imagery
P.O. Box 2070
Mill Valley, CA 94942
1-800-726-2070

If you are interested in learning more about naturopathic medicine, contact one of the naturopathic medical schools. Currently Bastyr University in Seattle, Washington, is the only fully accredited school that trains naturopathic physicians, although the National College of Naturopathic Medicine, in Portland, Oregon, is currently a candidate for accreditation. There is also a new school, in Scottsdale, Arizona, the Southwest College of Naturopathic Medicine. All colleges offer a four-year doctorate program leading to the Doctor of Naturopathic Medicine (N.D.) degree. Preadmission requirements at both schools are similar to conventional medical schools. For more information, contact:

Bastyr University
144 N.E. 54th St.
Seattle, WA 98105
(206) 523-9585

Southwest College of Naturopathic Medicine
10615 N. Hayden
Scottsdale, AZ
(602) 998-0323

National College of Naturopathic Medicine
11231 S.E. Market St.
Portland, OR 97216
(503) 255-4860

References

Introduction

1. Wortis, J., and Stone, A. The addiction to drug companies. *Biol. Psychiatry* 32:847–9, 1992.

Chapter 1: The Prozac Phenomenon

1. Stokes, P. E.: Fluoxetine. A five-year review. *Clinical Therapeutics* 15: 217–43, 1993; Gram, L. F.: Fluoxetine. *New Eng. J. Med.* 331: 1354–61, 1994.
2. Pande, A. C., and Sayler, M. E. Adverse events and treatment discontinuations in fluoxetine clinical trials. *Int. J. Psychopharmacol.* 8: 267–69, 1993.
3. Balon, R., et al. Sexual dysfunction during antidepressant treatment. *J. Clin. Psychiatry* 54:209–12, 1993.

References

Herman, M., and Goldbloom, D. S. Fluoxetine-induced sexual dysfunction. *J. Clin. Psychiatry* 42:25–27, 1990.

4. King, R. A., Segman, R. H., and Anderson, G. M. Serotonin and suicidality. The impact of acute fluoxetine administration. *Isr. J. Psychiatry Relat. Sci.* 31:271–79, 1994.

Tollefson, G. D., et al. Evaluation of suicidality during pharmacologic treatment of mood and nomood disorders. *Annals Clin. Psychology* 5:209–24, 1993.

Power, A. C., and Cowen, P. J. Fluoxetine and suicidal behaviour. *Br. J. Psychiatry* 161:735–41, 1992.

5. Wirshing, W. C., et al. Fluoxetine, akathisia and suicidality: is there a causal connection? *Archives Gen. Psychiatry* 49:580–81, 1992.

Creaney, W., Murray, I., and Healy, D. Antidepressant induced suicidal ideation. *Human Psychopharmacol.* 6:329–32, 1991.

Masand, P., Gupta, S., and Dewan, M. Suicidal ideation related to fluoxetine (letter). *New Eng. J. Med.* 324:420, 1991.

Rothschild, A. J., and Locke, C. A. Re-exposure to fluoxetine after serious suicide attempts by three patients: the role of akathisia. *J. Clin. Psychiatry* 52:491–93, 1991.

Dasgupta, K. Additional cases of suicidal ideation associated with fluoxetine (letter). *Am. J. Psychiatry* 147:1570, 1990.

Teicher, M. H., Glod, C., and Cole, J. O. Emergence of intense suicidal preoccupation during fluoxetine treatment. *Am. J. Psychiatry* 147:207–210, 1990.

6. Null, G. Prozac, Eli Lilly and the FDA. *Townsend Letter* #115/116: 134, 178–87, 1993.

7. Brandes, L. J., et al. Stimulation of malignant growth in rodents by antidepressant drugs at clinically relevant doses. *Cancer Res.* 52: 3,796–800, 1992.

8. Olfson, M., and Klerman, G. L. Trends in the prescription of antidepressants by office-based psychiatrists. *Am. J. Psychiatry* 150:571–77, 1993.

9. Olfson, M., and Pincus, H. A. Outpatient psychotherapy in the

United States, I: Volume, costs, and user characteristics. *Am. J. Psychiatry* 151:1281–88, 1994.

10. Rogers, W. H., et al. Outcomes for adult outpatients with depression under prepaid or fee-for-service financing. *Arch. Gen. Psychiatry* 50: 517–25, 1993.

Chapter 2: A Different View of Depression

1. Wetterberg, L. The relationship between the pineal gland and the pituitary-adrenal axis in health, endocrine and psychiatric conditions. *Psychoneuroendocrinology* 8:75–80, 1983.

    Miles, A., and Philbrick, D.R.S. Melatonin and psychiatry. *Biol. Psychiatry* 23:405–25, 1988.

2. Rosenthal, N., et al. Antidepressant effects of light in seasonal affective disorders. *Am. J. Psychiatry* 142:163–70, 1985.

    Rosenthal, N., et al. Seasonal affective disorder: a description of the syndrome and preliminary findings with light treatment. *Arch. Gen. Psychiatry* 41:72–80, 1984.

    Kripke, D., Risch, S., and Janowsky, D. Bright white light alleviates depression. *Psychiatric Res.* 10:105–12, 1983.

3. Martinez, B., et al. Hypericum in the treatment of seasonal affective disorders. *J. Geriatr. Psychiatry Neurol.* 7(Suppl 1):S29–33, 1994.

4. Peterson, C., Seligman, M., and Valliant, G. Pessimistic explanatory style as a risk factor for physical illness: A thirty-five-year longitudinal study. *J. Person. Soc. Psych.* 55:23–27, 1988.

    Peterson, C. Explanatory style as a risk factor for illness. *Cognitive Therapy and Research* 12:117–30, 1988.

5. Liparulo, R. Optimists can juice up your company's profit. *Real Estate Today* 28:12(5), 1995.

6. Jarrett, R. B., and Rush, A. J. Short-term psychotherapy of depressive disorders: current status and future directions. *Psychiatry* 57:115–32, 1994.

    Robins, C. J., and Hayes, A. M. An appraisal of cognitive

therapy. *J. Consult. Clin. Psychol.* 61:205–14, 1993.

7. Evans, M., et al. Differential relapse following cognitive therapy and pharmacotherapy for depression. *Arch. Gen. Psychiatry* 49:802–808, 1992.

Chapter 3: Ruling Out an Organic Cause

1. Nader, S. Premenstrual syndrome. *Postgraduate Med.* 90:173–80, 1991.

    Smith, S., and Schiff: The premenstrual syndrome—diagnosis and management. *Fertility Sterility* 52:527–43, 1989.

2. Abraham, G. E. Nutritional factors in the etiology of the premenstrual tension syndromes. *J. Repro. Med.* 28:446–64, 1983.

3. Rossignol, A. M., and Bonnlander, H. Prevalence and severity of the premenstrual syndrome. Effects of foods and beverages that are sweet or high in sugar content. *J. Reprod. Med.* 36:132–36, 1991.

4. London, R. S., Bradley, L., and Chiamori, N. Y. Effect of a nutritional supplement on premenstrual symptomatology in women with premenstrual syndrome: A double-blind longitudinal study. *J. Am. Coll. Nutr.* 10:494–9, 1991.

    Goei, G. S., and Abraham, G. E. Effect of nutritional supplement, Optivite, on symptoms of premenstrual tension. *J. Repro. Med.* 28:527–31, 1983.

5. Abraham, G. E., and Hargrove, J. T. Effect of vitamin B6 on premenstrual symptomatology in women with premenstrual tension syndromes: A double-blind crossover study. *Infert.* 3:155–65, 1980.

6. Facchinetti, F., et al. Oral magnesium successfully relieves premenstrual mood changes. *Obstet. Gynecol.* 78:177–81, 1991.

7. Holmes, T. H., and Rahe, R. H. The social readjustment scale. *J. Psychosomatic Res.* 11:213–18, 1967.

8. Carroll, B. J., Curtis, G. C., and Mendels, J. Cerebrospinal fluid and plasma free cortisol concentrations in depression. *Psychol. Med.* 6:235–44, 1976.

References

9. Altar, C., et al. Glucocorticoid induction of tryptophan oxygenase. *Biochem. Pharmacol.* 32:979–84, 1983.

10. Hikino, H. Traditional remedies and modern assessment: The case of ginseng. In *The Medicinal Plant Industry*. Wijeskera, R.O.B. (ed.). CRC Press, Boca Raton, Fla., 1991, chap. 11, pp. 149–66.

    Shibata, S., et al. Chemistry and pharmacology of Panax. *Econ. Med. Plant Research* 1:217–84, 1985.

11. Schottenfeld, R. S., and Cullen, M. R. Organic affective illness associated with lead intoxication. *Am. J. Psychiatry* 141:1423–26, 1984.

    Rutter, M., and Russell-Jones, R. (eds.). *Lead Versus Health: Sources and Effects of Low Level Lead Exposure*. John Wiley, New York, 1983.

    Seaton, A., Jeelinek, E. H., and Kennedy, P. Major neurological disease and occupational exposure to organic solvents. *Quart. J. Med.* 305:707–12, 1992.

12. Rowe, A. H., and Rowe, A , Jr. *Food Allergy. Its Manifestations and Control and the Elimination Diets. A Compendium*. Charles C. Thomas, Springfield, Ill., 1972.

13. Brostoff, J., and Challacombe, S. J. (eds.). *Food Allergy and Intolerance*. W. B. Saunders, Philadelphia, 1987.

14. Gold, M., Pottash, A., and Extein, I. Hypothyroidism and depression, evidence from complete thyroid function evaluation. *J. Amonoamine* 245:1919–22, 1981.

    Joffe, R., Roy-Byrne, P., and Udhe, T. Thyroid function and affective illness: a reappraisal. *Biol. Psychiatry* 19:1685–91, 1984.

15. Barnes, B. O., and Galton, L. *Hypothyroidism: The Unsuspected Illness*. Thomas Crowell, New York, 1976.

    Langer, S. E., and Scheer, J. F. *Solved: The Riddle of Illness*. Keats, New Canaan, Conn., 1984.

16. Winokur, A., et al. Insulin resistance after glucose tolerance testing in patients with major depression. *Am. J. Psychiatry* 145:325–30, 1988.

    Wright, J. H., Jacisin, J. J., Radin, N. S., et al. Glucose metabolism in unipolar depression. *Br. J. Psychiatry* 132:386–93, 1978.

17. Hadji-Georgopoulus, A., et al. Elevated hypoglycemic index and late hyperinsulinism in symptomatic postprandial hypoglycemia. *J. Clin. Endocrinol. Metabol.* 50:371–76, 1980.

Fabrykant, M. The problem of functional hyperinsulinism on functional hypoglycemia attributed to nervous causes. 1. Laboratory and clinical correlations. *Metabolism* 4:469–79, 1955.

Chapter 4: Lifestyle Factors in Depression

1. Beasley, J. *The Betrayal of Health. The Impact of Nutrition, Environment, and Lifestyle on Illness in America.* Random House, New York, 1991.

2. Fielding, J. E. Smoking: health effects and control. *New Eng. J. Med.* 313:491–98, 555–61, 1985.

Mattson, M. E., Pollack, E. S., and Cullen, J. W. What are the odds smoking will kill you? *Am. J. Publ. Health* 77:425–31, 1987.

3. Kinsman, R., and Hood, J. Some behavioral effects of ascorbic acid deficiency. *Am. J. Clin. Nutr.* 24:455–64, 1971.

4. Chou, T. Wake up and smell the coffee. Caffeine, coffee, and the medical consequences. *West. J. Med.* 157:544–53, 1992.

Niems, A., and von Borstel, R. Caffeine: metabolism and biochemical mechanisms of action. In: *Nutrition and the Brain,* vol. 6. Wurtman, R., and Wurtman, J. (eds.). Raven Press, New York, 1983, pp. 2–30.

5. Gilliand, K., and Bullick, W. Caffeine: A potential drug of abuse. *Adv. Alcohol Subst. Abuse* 3:53–73, 1984.

6. Greden, J., et al. Anxiety and depression associated with caffeinism among psychiatric patients. *Am. J. Psychiatry* 131:1089–94, 1979.

Neil, J. F., et al. Caffeinism complicating hypersomnic depressive disorders. *Compr. Psychiatry* 19:377–85, 1978.

7. Charney, D., Henninger, G., and Jatlow, P. Increased anxiogenic effects of caffeine in panic disorders. *Arch. Gen. Psychiatry* 42:233–43, 1984.

References

Bolton, S., and Null, G. Caffeine, psychological effects, use and abuse. *J. Orthomol. Psychiatry* 10:202–11, 1981.

8. Kreitsch, K., et al. Prevalence, presenting symptoms, and psychological characteristics of individuals experiencing a diet-related mood disturbance. *Behav. Ther.* 19:593–94, 1985.

9. Christensen, L. Psychological distress and diet—effects of sucrose and caffeine. *J. Apl. Nutr.* 40:44–50, 1988.

10. Martin, J. E., and Dubbert, P. M. Exercise applications and promotion in behavioral medicine. *J. Consult. Clin. Psychol.* 50:1004–17, 1982.

11. Weyerer, S., and Kupfer, B. Physical exercise and psychological health. *Sports Med.* 17:108–16, 1994.

12. Carr, D., et al. Physical conditioning facilitates the exercise-induced secretion of beta-endorphin and beta-lipoprotein in women. *New Eng. J. Med.* 305:560–65, 1981.

13. Lobstein, D., Mosbacher, B. J., and Ismail, A. H. Depression as a powerful discriminator between physically active and sedentary middle-aged men. *J. Psychosom. Res.* 27:69–76, 1983.

14. Folkins, C. H., and Sime, W. E. Physical fitness training and mental health. *Am. Psychologist* 36:375–88, 1981.

15. Martinsen, E. W. The role of aerobic exercise in the treatment of depression. *Stress Med.* 3:93–100, 1987.

16. Weyerer, S., and Kupfer, B. Physical exercise and psychological health. *Sports Med.* 17:108–16, 1994.

Byrne, A., and Byrne, D. G. The effect of exercise on depression, anxiety and other mood states: a review. *J. Psychosom. Res.* 37:565–74, 1993.

Koeppl, P. M., et al. The influence of weight reduction and exercise regimes upon the personality profiles of overweight males. *J. Clin. Psychol.* 48:463–71, 1992.

Dua, J., and Hargreaves, L. Effect of aerobic exercise on negative affect, positive affect, stress, and depression. *Percept. Mot. Skills* 75: 355–61, 1992.

Stein, P. N., and Motta, R. W. Effects of aerobic and nonaerobic exercise on depression and self-concept. *Percept. Mot. Skills* 74:79–89, 1992.

   Casper, R. C. Exercise and mood. *World Rev. Nutr. Diet* 71:115–43, 1993.

   LaFontaine, T. P., et al. Aerobic exercise and mood. A brief review, 1985–1990. *Sports Med.* 13:160–70, 1992.

   Steege, J. F., and Blumenthal, J. A. The effects of aerobic exercise on premenstrual symptoms in middle-aged women: a preliminary study. *J. Psychosom. Res.* 37(2):127–33, 1993.

17. Smith, W. P., Compton, W. C., and West, W. B. Meditation as an adjunct to a happiness enhancement program. *J. Clin. Psychol.* 51:269–73, 1995.

18. Richman, J. The lifesaving function of humor with the depressed and suicidal elderly. *Gerontologist* 35:271–73, 1995.

19. Fry, W. F., Jr. The physiologic effects of humor, mirth, and laughter. *J. Amonoamine* 267:1857–58, 1992.

Chapter 5: Nutritional Factors in Depression

1. Werbach, M. *Nutritional Influences on Mental Illness: A Sourcebook of Clinical Research.* Third Line Press, Tarzana, Calif., 1991.

2. Stanto, J. L., and Keast, D. R. Serum cholesterol, fat intake, and breakfast consumption in the United States adult population. *J. Am. Coll. Nutr.* 8:567–72, 1989.

3. National Research Council. *Diet and Health. Implications for Reducing Chronic Disease Risk.* National Academy Press, Washington, D.C., 1989.

4. National Research Council. *Recommended Dietary Allowances,* 10th ed. National Academy Press, Washington, D.C., 1989.

5. Crellin, R., Bottiglieri, T., and Reynolds, E. H. Folates and psychiatric disorders. Clinical potential. *Drugs* 45:623–36, 1993.

   Carney, M.W.P., et al. Red cell folate concentrations in

References

psychiatric patients. *J. Affective Disorders* 19:207–13, 1990.

Godfrey, P.S.A., et al. Enhancement of recovery from psychiatric illness by methy folate. *Lancet* 336:392–95, 1990.

Reynolds, E., et al. Folate deficiency in depressive illness. *Br. J. Psychiatry* 117:287–92, 1970.

6. Thornton, W. E., and Thornton, B. P. Geriatric mental function and folic acid: A review and survey. *Southern Med. J.* 70:919–22, 1977.

Abalan, F., et al. Frequency of deficiencies of vitamin B_{12} and folic acid in patients admitted to a geriatric-psychiatry unit. *Encephale* 10:9–12, 1984.

7. Zucker, D., et al. B_{12} deficiency and psychiatric disorders: a case report and literature review. *Biol Psychiatry* 16:197–205, 1981.

Kivela, S. L., Pahkala, K., and Eronen, A. Depression in the aged: Relation to folate and vitamins C and B_{12}. *Biol. Psychiatry* 26:209–13, 1989.

8. Curtius, H., Muldner, H., and Niederwieser, A. Tetrahydrobiopterin: Efficacy in endogenous depression and Parkinson's disease. *J. Neural. Trans.* 55:301–308, 1982.

Curtius, H., et al. Successful treatment of depression with tetrahydrobiopterin. *Lancet* i:657–58, 1983.

9. Leeming, R., et al. Tetrahydrofolate and hydroxycobolamin in the management of Dihydropteridine reductase deficiency. *J. Ment. Def. Res.* 26:21–25, 1982.

10. Botez, M., et al. Effect of folic acid and vitamin B_{12} deficiencies on 5-hydroxyindoleacetic acid in human cerebrospinal fluid. *Ann. Neurol.* 12:479–84, 1982.

Reynolds, E., and Stramentinoli, G. Folic acid, S-adenosylmethionine and affective disorder. *Psychol. Med.* 13:705–10, 1983.

Reynolds, E., Carney, M., and Toone, B. Methylation and mood. *Lancet* ii:196–99, 1983.

11. Crellin, R., Bottiglieri, T., and Reynolds, E. H. Folates and psychiatric disorders. Clinical potential. *Drugs* 45:623–36, 1993.

12. Russ, C., Hendricks, T., Chrisley, B., Kalin, N., and Driskell, J.

Vitamin B$_6$ status of depressed and obsessive-compulsive patients. *Nutr. Rep. Intl.* 27:867–73, 1983.

Carney, M., Williams, D., and Sheffield, B. Thiamin and pyridoxine lack in newly-admitted psychiatric patients. *Br. J. Psychiatry* 135:249–54, 1979.

Nobbs, B. Pyridoxal phosphate status in clinical depression. *Lancet* i:405, 1974.

Stewart, J. W., Harrison, W., Quitkin, F., and Baker, H. Low level B$_6$ levels in depressed outpatients. *Biolog. Psychiat.* 19:613–16, 1984.

13. Simopoulos, A. P. Omega-3 fatty acids in health and disease and in growth and development. *Am. J. Clin. Nutr.* 54:438–63, 1991.

Bjerve, K. S., et al. Clinical studies with alpha-linolenic acid and long chain n-3 fatty acids. *Nutrition* 8:130–32, 1992.

Bougnoix, P., et al. Alpha-linolenic acid content of adipose breast tissue: A host determinant of the risk of early metastasis in breast cancer. *Br. J. Cancer* 70:330–34, 1994.

Rose, D. P., and Hatala, M. Dietary fatty acids and breast cancer invasion and metastasis. *Nutr. Cancer* 21:103–11, 1994.

14. Hibbeln, J. R., and Salem, N. Dietary polyunsaturated fatty acids and depression: when cholesterol does not satisfy. *Am. J. Clin. Nutr.* 62:1–9, 1995.

Chapter 6: St. John's Wort Extract

1. Morazzoni, P., and Bombardelli, E. Hypericum perforatum. *Fitoterapia* 66:43–68, 1995.

Harrer, G., and Schulz, V. Clinical investigation of the antidepressant effectiveness of Hypericum. *J. Geriatr. Psychiatry Neurol.* 7(Suppl 1):S6–8, 1994.

2. Sommer, H., and Harrer, G. Placebo-controlled double-blind study examining the effectiveness of an hypericum preparation in 105

mildly depressed patients. *J. Geriatr. Psychiatry Neurol.* 7(Suppl 1): S9–11, 1994.

3. Harrer, G., and Sommer, H. Treatment of mild/moderate depressions with Hypericum. *Phytomed.* 1:3–8, 1994.

Hoffmann, J., and Kuhl, E. D. Treatment of depressive conditions with hypericin. *Z. Allgemeinmed.* 12:776–82, 1979.

Schlich, D., Brauckmann, F., and Schenk, N. Treatment of depressive conditions with hypericum. *Psychol.* 13:440–44, 1987.

Halama, P. Efficacy of the Hypericum extract LI 160 in the treatment of 50 patients of a psychiatrist. *Nervenheilkunde* 10:305–307, 1991.

Panijel, M. Treatment of moderate states of anxiety. *Therapiewoche* 41:4,659–68, 1985.

Schmidt, U., et al. The therapy of depressive moods. *Psycho.* 15: 665–71, 1989.

Schmidt, U., and Sommer, H. St. John's wort extract in the ambulatory therapy of depression. Attention and reaction ability are preserved. *Fortschr. Med.* 111:339–42, 1993.

Steger, W. Depressive moods. *Z. Allgemeinmed.* 61:914–18, 1985.

4. Vorbach, E. U., Hubner, W. D., and Arnoldt, K. H. Effectiveness and tolerance of the hypericum extract LI 160 in comparison with imipramine: randomized double-blind study with 135 outpatients. *J. Geriatr. Psychiatry Neurol.* 7(Suppl 1):S19–23, 1994.

5. Harrer, G., Hubner, W. D., and Podzuweit, H. Effectiveness and tolerance of the hypericum extract LI 160 compared to maprotiline: a multicenter double-blind study. *J. Geriatr. Psychiatry Neurol.* 7(Suppl 1):S24–28, 1994.

6. Johnson, D., et al. Effects of hypericum extract LI 160 compared with maprotiline on resting EEG and evoked potentials in 24 volunteers. *J. Geriatr. Psychiatry Neurol.* 7(Suppl 1):S44–46, 1994.

7. Schulz, H., and Jobert, M. Effects of hypericum extract on the sleep EEG in older volunteers. *J. Geriatr. Psychiatry Neurol.* 7(Suppl 1): S39–43, 1994.

8. Bladt, S., and Wagner, H. Inhibition of monoamineO by fractions and constituents of hypericum extract. *J. Geriatr. Psychiatry Neurol.* 7(Suppl 1):S57–59, 1994.

    Thiede, H. M., and Walper, A. Inhibition of monoamineO and COMT by hypericum extracts and hypericin. *J. Geriatr. Psychiatry Neurol.* 7(Suppl 1):S54–56, 1994.

    Suzuki, O., et al. Inhibition of monoamine oxidase by hypericin. *Planta Medica* 50:272–74, 1984.

    Holzl, J., Demisch, L., and Gollnik, B. Investigations about antidepressive and mood changing effects of Hypericum perforatum. *Planta Medica* 55:643, 1989.

9. Muldner, V. H., and Zoller, M. Antidepressive wirkung eines auf den wirkstoffkomplex hypericin standardisierten hypericumextrakes. *Arzneim Forsch.* 34:918, 1984.

10. Woelk, H., Burkard, G., and Grunwald, J. Benefits and risks of the hypericum extract LI 160: drug monitoring study with 3250 patients. *J. Geriatr. Psychiatry Neurol.* 7(Suppl 1):S34–38, 1994.

Chapter 7: Kava Extract

1. Lebot, V., Merlin, M., and Lindstrom, L. *Kava. The Pacific Drug.* Yale University Press, New Haven, 1992.

    Singh, Y.: Kava. An overview. *J. Ethnopharmacol.* 37:13–45, 1992.

2. Meyer, H. J. Pharmacology of Kava. In: *Ethnopharmacological Search for Psychoactive Drugs.* Holmstedt, B., and Kline, N. S. (eds.). Raven Press, New York, 1979, pp. 133–40.

3. Keledjian, J., et al. Uptake into mouse brain of four compounds present in the psychoactive beverage kava. *J. Pharm. Sci.* 77:1003–1006, 1988.

4. Davies, L. P., et al. Kava pyrones and resin: Studies on GABAa, GABAb and benzodiazepine binding sites in rodent brain. *Pharm. Toxicol.* 71:120–26, 1992.

References

5. Scholing, W. E., and Clausen, H. D. On the effect of d,l-kavain: experience with neuronika. *Med. Klin.* 72:1301–306, 1977.

6. Lindenberg, D., and Pitule-Schodel, H. D,L-kavain in comparison with oxazepam in anxiety disorders. A double-blind study of clinical effectiveness. *Forschr. Med.* 108:49–50, 53–54, 1990.

7. Kinzler, E., Kromer, J., and Lehmann, E. Clinical efficacy of a kava extract in patients with anxiety syndrome: double-blind placebo controlled study over 4 weeks. *Arzneim Forsch.* 41:584–88, 1991.

8. Warnecke, G. Neurovegetative dystonia in the female climacteric. Studies on the clinical efficacy and tolerance of kava extract WS 1490. *Fortschr. Med.* 109:120–22, 1991.

9. Herberg, K. W. The influence of kava–special extract WS 1490 on safety-relevant performance alone and in combination with ethyl-alcohol. *Blutalkohol* 30:96–105, 1993.

10. Munte, T. F., et al. Effects of oxazepam and an extract of kava roots (*Piper methysticum*) on event-related potentials in a word recognition task. *Neuropsychobiol.* 27:46–53, 1993.

11. Holm, E., et al. Studies on the profile of the neurophysiological effects of D,L-kavain: cerebral sites of action and sleep-wakefulness-rhythm in animals. *Arzneim Forsch.* 41:673–83, 1991.

12. Jamieson, D. D., and Duffield, P. H. The antinociceptive action of kava components in mice. *Clin. Exp. Pharmacol. Physiol.* 17:495–508, 1990.

13. Duffield, P. H., and Jamieson, D. Development of tolerance to kava in mice. *Clin. Exp. Pharmacol. Physiol.* 18:571–78, 1991.

14. Schelosky, L., et al. Kava and dopamine antagonism [letter]. *J. Neurol. Neurosurg. Psychiatry* 58:639–40, 1995.

15. Norton, S. A., and Ruze, P.: Kava dermopathy. *J. Am. Acad. Dermatol.* 31:89–97, 1994.

16. Ruze, P.: Kava-induced dermopathy. a niacin deficiency. *Lancet* 335:1442–45, 1990.

17. Mathews, J. D., et al. Effects of the heavy usage of kava on physical health: summary of a pilot survey in an Aboriginal community. *Med. J. Aust.* 148:548–55, 1988.

Chapter 8: Ginkgo Biloba Extract

1. DeFeudis, F. V. (ed.). *Ginkgo Biloba Extract (EGb 761). Pharmacological Activities and Clinical Applications.* Paris, Elsevier, 1991.

   Funfgeld, E. W. (ed.). *Rokan (Ginkgo Biloba). Recent Results in Pharmacology and Clinic.* Springer-Verlag, New York, 1988.

   Kleijnen, J., and Knipschild, P. Ginkgo biloba. *Lancet* 340:1136–39, 1992.

2. Kleijnen, J., and Knipschild, P. Ginkgo biloba for cerebral insufficiency. *Br. J. Clinical Pharmacol.* 34:352–58, 1992.

3. Hansgen, K. D., Vesper, J., and Ploch, M. Multicenter double-blind study examining the antidepressant effectiveness of the hypericum extract LI 160. *J. Geriatr. Psychiatry Neurol.* 7(Suppl 1):S15–18, 1994.

   Hubner, W. D., Lande, S., and Podzuweit, H. Hypericum treatment of mild depressions with somatic symptoms. *J. Geriatr. Psychiatry Neurol.* 7(Suppl 1):S12–14, 1994.

   Schmidt, U., Rabinovici, K., and Lande, S. Einfluss eines Ginkgo biloba specialextraktes auf doe befomdlickeit bei zerebraler onsufficizienz. *Munch. Med. Wockenschr.* 133(suppl. 1):S15–18, 1991.

   Bruchert, E., Heinrich, S. E., and Ruf-Kohler, P. Wirksamkeit von LI 1370 bei alteren patienten mit himleistungsschwache. Multizentrische doppelblindstudie des fachverbandes Deutscher Allegemeinaezte. *Munch. Med. Wockenschr.* 133(suppl. 1):S9–14, 1991.

   Meyer, B. Etude multicentrique randomisee a double insu face au placebo due traitment des acouphenes par l'extrait de Ginkgo biloba. *Presse Med* 15:1562–64, 1986.

   Taillandier, J., et al. Traitment des troubles du vidillissement cerebral pal l'extrait Ginkgo biloba. *Presse Med* 15:1583–87, 1986.

   Haguenauer, J. P., et al. Traitment des troubles de l'equilibre par l'extrait Ginkgo biloba. *Presse Med.* 15:1569–72, 1986.

References

Vorberg, G., Schmidt, U., and Schenk, N. Wirksamkeit eines neuen Ginkgo biloba extraktes bei 100 patienten mit zerebraler insuffizienz. *Herg Gefasse* 9:936–41, 1989.

Eckmann, F. Himleistungsstorungen: Behandlung mit Ginkgo biloba extrakt. *Forsch. Med.* 108:557–60, 1990.

Wesnes, K., et al. A double-blind placebo-controlled trial of Tanakan in the treatment of idiopathic cognitive impairment in the elderly. *Hum. Psychopharmacol.* 2:159–69, 1987.

4. Anadere, I., Chmiel, H., and Witte, S. Hemorrheological findings in patients with completed stroke and the influence of Ginkgo biloba extract. *Clin. Hemorheo.* 4:411–20, 1985.

5. Gessner, B., Voelp, A., and Klasser, M. Study of the long-term action of a Ginkgo biloba extract on vigilance and mental performance as determined by means of quantitative pharmaco-EEG and psychometric measurements. *Arzneim Forsch.* 35:1459–65, 1985.

Hofferberth, B. Effect of Ginkgo biloba extract on neurophysiological and psychometric measurement in patients with cerebroorganic syndrome. A double-blind study versus placebo. *Arzneim Forsch.* 39:918–22, 1989.

6. Hindmarch, I., and Subhan, Z. The psychopharmacological effects of Ginkgo biloba extract in normal healthy volunteers. *Int. J. Clin. Pharmacol. Res.* 4:89–93, 1984.

7. Schubert, H., and Halama, P. Depressive episode primarily unresponsive to therapy in elderly patients: Efficacy of Ginkgo biloba (Egb 761) in combination with antidepressants. *Geriatr. Forsch.* 3: 45–53, 1993.

8. Huguet, F., et al. Decreased cerebral 5-HT_{1a} receptors during aging: reversal by Ginkgo biloba extract (Egb 761). *J. Pharm. Pharmacol.* 46:316–18, 1994.

9. Becker, L. E., and Skipworth, G. B. Ginkgo-tree dermatitis, stomatitis, and proctitis. *J. Amonoamine* 231:1162–63, 1975.

10. Hofferberth, B. The efficacy of Egb761 in patients with senile dementia of the Alzheimer type. A double-blind, placebo-controlled

study on different levels of investigation. *Human Psychopharmacol.* 9: 215–22, 1994.

11. Engel, R. R., et al. Double-blind cross-over study of phosphatidyl-serine vs. placebo in patients with early dementia of the Alzheimer type. *Eur. Neuropsychopharmacol.* 2:149–55, 1992.

12. Cenacchi, T., et al. Cognitive decline in the elderly: a double-blind, placebo-controlled multicenter study on efficacy of phosphatidyl-serine administration. *Aging* 5:123–33, 1993.

Crook, T., et al. Effects of phosphatidylserine in Alzheimer's disease. *Psychopharmacol. Bull.* 28:61–66, 1992.

Crook, T. H., et al. Effects of phosphatidylserine in age-associated memory impairment. *Neurology* 41:644–49, 1991.

Funfgeld, E. W., et al. Double-blind study with phosphatidyl-serine (PS) in parkinsonian patients with senile dementia of Alzheimer's type (SDAT). *Prog. Clin. Biol. Res.* 317:1235–46, 1989.

13. Maggioni, M., et al. Effects of phosphatidylserine therapy in geriatric patients with depressive disorders. *Acta Psychiatr. Scand.* 81:265–70, 1990.

14. Monteleone, P., et al. Effects of phosphatidylserine on the neuroen-docrine response to physical stress in humans. *Neuroendocrinology* 52: 243–48, 1990.

Monteleone, P., et al. Blunting chronic phosphatidylserine ad-ministration of the stress-induced activation of the hypothalamo-pituitary-adrenal axis in healthy men. *Eur. J. Clin. Pharamacol.* 41: 385–88, 1992.

Nerozzi, D., et al. Early cortisol escape phenomenon reversed by phosphatidylserine in elderly normal subjects. *Clinical Trial J.* 26: 33–38, 1989.

Chapter 9: Amino Acids

1. Slutsker, L., et al. Eosinophilia-myalgia syndrome associated with ex-posure to tryptophan from a single manufacturer. *JAMA* 264:213–17, 1990.

References

Belongia, E. A., et al. An investigation of the cause of the eosinophilia-myalgia syndrome associated with tryptophan use. *New Eng. J. Med.* 323:357–65, 1990.

Kaufman, L. D., and Philen, R. M. Tryptophan. Current status and future trends for oral administration. *Drug Safety* 8:89–98, 1993.

2. Brown, R. Tryptophan metabolism in humans. In: *Biochemical and Medical Aspects of Tryptophan Metabolism.* Hayaishi, O., Ishimura, Y., and Kido, R. (eds.). Elsevier/North Holland Press, Amsterdam, 1980, pp. 227–36.

3. Boman, B. L-tryptophan: A rational antidepressant and a natural hypnotic? *Aust. N.Z.J. Psychiatry* 22:83–97, 1988.

Chouinard, G., et al. Tryptophan in the treatment of depression and mania. *Adv. Biol. Psychiatry* 10:47–66, 1983.

Gibson, C. Control of monoamine synthesis by amino acid precursors. *Adv. Biol. Psychiatry* 10:4–18, 1983.

Moller, S., Kirk, L., Brandrup, E., et al. Tryptophan availability in endogenous depression—relation to efficacy of L-tryptophan treatment. *Adv. Biol. Psychiatry* 10:30–46, 1983.

4. Beckman, H. Phenylalanine in affective disorders. *Adv. Biol. Psychiatry* 10:137–47, 1983.

Gibson, C., and Gelenberg, A. Tyrosine for depression. *Adv. Biol. Psychiatry* 10:148–59, 1983.

5. Baldessarini, R. J. Neuropharmacology of S-adenosyl-L-methionine. *Am. J. Med.* 83(Suppl.5A):95–103, 1987.

Reynolds, E., Carney, M., and Toone, B. Methylation and mood. *Lancet* ii:196–99, 1983.

Bottiglieri, T., Laundry, M., Martin, R., et al. S-adenosylmethionine influences monoamine metabolism. *Lancet* ii: 224, 1984.

6. Janicak P. G., et al. Parenteral S-adenosylmethionine in depression. A literature review and preliminary report. *Psychopharmacol. Bull.* 25:238–41, 1989.

Friedel, H. A., Goa, K. L., and Benfield, P. S-adenosylmethionine. *Drugs* 38:3,389–417, 1989.

Carney, M.W.P., Toone, B. K., and Reynolds, E. H. S-adenosylmethionine and affective disorder. *Am. J. Med.* 83(Suppl.5A):104–106, 1987.

Vahora, S. A., and Malek-Ahmadi, P. S-adenosylmethionine in depression. *Neurosci. Biobehav. Rev.* 12:139–41, 1988.

7. Kagan, B. L., et al. Oral S-adenosylmethionine in depression. A randomized, double-blind placebo-controlled trial. *Am. J. Psychiatry* 147:591–95, 1990.

Rosenbaum, J. F., et al. An open-label pilot study of oral S-adenosylmethionine in major depression. *Psychopharmacol. Bull.* 24: 189–94, 1988.

De Vanna, M., and Rigamonti, R. Oral S-adenosyl-L-methionine in depression. *Curr. Ther. Res.* 52:478–85, 1992.

Salmaggi, P., et al. Double-blind, placebo-controlled study of S-adenosyl-L-methionine in depressed postmenopausal women. *Psychother. Psychosom.* 59:34–40, 1993.

8. Bell, K. M., et al. S-adenosylmethionine blood levels in major depression: changes with drug treatment. *Acta Neurol. Scand.* 154(Suppl.):15–18, 1994.

9. Braverman, E., and Pfieffer, C. *The Healing Nutrients Within. Facts, Findings and New Research on Amino Acids.* Keats Publishing, New Canaan, Conn., 1987.

Chapter 10: Melatonin

1. Yu, H. S., and Reiter, R. J. (eds.) *Melatonin biosynthesis, physiological effects and clinical applications.* CRC Press, Boca Raton, Fla., 1993.

Waldhauser, F., Ehrhart, B., and Forster, E. Clinical aspects of the melatonin action. *Experentia* 49:671–81, 1993.

2. Arendt, J., et al. Some effects of jet-lag and their alleviation by melatonin. *Ergonomics* 30:1379–93, 1987.

Claustrat, B., et al. Melatonin and jet lag: Confirmatory result

References

using a simplified protocol. *Biol. Psychiatry* 32:705–11, 1992.

Petrie, K., et al. Effect of melatonin on jet lag after long haul flights. *Br. Med. J.* 298:705–7, 1989.

Lino, A., et al. Melatonin and jet lag: *Treatment schedule* 34:587, 1993.

3. Petrie, K., et al. A double-blind trial of melatonin as a treatment for jet lag in international cabin crew. *Biol. Psychiatry* 33:526–30, 1993.

4. Maurizi, C. Disorder of the pineal gland associated with depression, peptic ulcers, and sexual dysfunction. *Southern Med. J.* 77:1516–18, 1984.

Wetterberg, L. The relationship between the pineal gland and the pituitary-adrenal axis in health, endocrine and psychiatric conditions. *Psychoneuroendocrinology* 8:75–80, 1983.

Beck, F., et al. Serum melatonin in relation to clinical variables in patients with major depressive mood and a hypothesis of low melatonin syndrome. *Acta Psychiatr. Scand.* 71:319–30, 1985.

5. Rubin, R. L., et al. Neuroendocrine aspects of primary endogenous depression. XI. Serum melatonin measures in patients and matched control subjects. *Arch. Gen. Psychiat.* 49:558–67, 1992.

Thompson, C., et al. A comparison of melatonin secretion in depressed patients and normal subjects. *Br. J. Psychiatry* 152:260–65, 1988.

Waterman, G. S., et al. Nocturnal urinary excretion of 6-hydroxymelatonin sulfate in prepubertal major depressive disorder. *Biol. Psych.* 31:582–90, 1992.

6. Mallo, C., et al. Effects of a four-day nocturnal melatonin treatment on the 24 h plasma melatonin, cortisol and prolactin profiles in humans. *Acta Endocrinologia* 119:474–80, 1988.

7. Carman, J. S., et al. Negative effects of melatonin on depression. *Am. J. Psychiatry* 133:1181–86, 1976.

8. Dollins, A. B., et al. Effect of pharmacological daytime doses of melatonin on human mood and performance. *Psychopharmacology* 112:490–96, 1993.

9. Waldhauser, F., Saletu, B., and Trinchard-Lugan, I. Sleep laboratory

investigations on hypnotic properties of melatonin. *Psychopharmacology* 100:222–26, 1990.

Zhdanova, I. V., et al. Sleep-inducing effects of low doses of melatonin ingested in the evening. *Clin. Pharmacol. Ther.* 57:552–58, 1995.

Dahlitz, M., et al. Delayed sleep phase syndrome response to melatonin. *Lancet* 337:1121–24, 1991.

10. MacFarlane, J. G., et al. The effects of exogenous melatonin on the total sleep time and daytime alertness of chronic insomniacs: a preliminary study. *Biol. Psychiatry* 30:371–76, 1991.

James, S. P., et al. Melatonin administration in insomnia. *Neuropsychopharmacology* 3:19–23, 1990.

11. Nave, R., Peled, R., and Lavie, P. Melatonin improves evening napping. *Eur. J. Pharmacol.* 275:213–16, 1995.

12. Dollins, A. B., et al. Effect of inducing nocturnal serum melatonin concentrations in daytime on sleep, mood, body temperature, and performance. *Proc. Natl. Acad. Sci. USA* 91:1824–28, 1994.

13. Fellenberg, A. J., Phillipou, G., and Seamark, R. F. Measurement of urinary production rates of melatonin as an index of human pineal function. *Endocr. Res. Comm.* 7:167–75, 1980.

Chapter II: Putting It All Together

1. Leathwood, P., et al. Aqueous extract of valerian root (Valeriana officinalis L.) improves sleep quality in man. *Pharmacol. Biochem. Behavior* 17:65–71, 1982.

Leathwood, P. D., and Chauffard, F. Aqueous extract of valerian reduces latency to fall asleep in man. *Planta Medica* 54:144–48, 1985.

Lindahl, O., and Lindwall, L. Double-blind study of a valerian preparation. *Pharmacol. Biochem. Behavior* 32:1065–66, 1989.

Index

Index

Index

Index

Index

Index